= "Tara has put together a beautiful collectic.. .. .... ...... assisted and unassisted birth stories. She also shares her thoughts on how to achieve an unhindered birth. I highly recommend it."
-- Laura Shanley

= "Great book. I haven't finished reading it yet, but I love the stories about her births, her surrogacy and UC, and the other stories that are just so real and un-sugar-coated. Once I get caught up I'm going to finish it and post my own review, but this is just too good to pass up!"
-- Unassisted Birth/Freebirth

= "Your burst of confidence and wisdom was exactly what I needed... I birthed my breech baby in water at my midwife's home about 16 hours after receiving your encouragement! I am woman... hear me ROAR!"
-- Julie Orris Kosker

= "Tara has a gift for empowering people to access their innate personal power and wisdom. Her expertise, confidence, and ease is magnetic and reassuring."
-- Dr. Zohra Campbell, D.C.

= "Reading Birth Unhindered will move women towards making informed decisions that will impact their birth experience by replacing fear with knowledge thus increasing confidence. This leads towards a positive birth experience."
-- Carol Severson LDM,CPM,CMA

= "Birth Unhindered will inspire women to believe in themselves and what their body was made to do."

-- Brandi McDaniel, home-schooling mother of three.


= "When you meet Tara in her writing, you have an instant friend who walks you through the practical steps of the pregnancy and birthing process. Tara is able to, in a fun and entertaining way, teach me fundamentals I thought I knew. Birth Unhindered will guide you with tips, tools, and techniques helpful to have a joyful pregnancy and birth experience. This book has helped me and my practice 110%. Thank you, Tara!"

-- Ryan Kackley, Celt System Founder,  Relationship Consulting, N.L.P. C.Ht. E.F.T

# Birth

# Unhindered

## By Tara L. McGuire

Professional photos of Tara L. McGuire by:

•Gregory Dean Design

International Standard Book Number (ISBN)

978-0-9845942-0-7


Library of Congress Control Number (LCCN)

2010932258

# Dedication

This book is dedicated first, and foremost to my children; Austin, for teaching me that life is about love, patience, and service. Jonah, for teaching me that releasing our expectations is healthy, at times. My lost babies for teaching me to yearn, grieve, and mourn. Faith for teaching me the power of believing in what we cannot see or feel. Grace for teaching me that there is a time for fullness in all endeavors. Mikayla for teaching me how beautifully pain and love can intermingle.

I would like to thank the dear women who shared their intimate and vulnerable moments along with their moments of joy, pain, weakness and strength with us in this book. Without them, this would not be. I am honored by their contributions and like-minded desire to influence and empower other women.

It would be negligent to not thank my mother and father for not only giving me life, but always loving me and believing in me.

Most deservedly, I thank the love of my life; Don. You are truly the wind beneath my wings. The solid ground when I need, and the song in my ear, always. I will cherish every day of our lives together. Without you, I wouldn't be me.

# Contents (chapters)

# Preface

It is my dream and intention that birthing mothers and fathers might read this book and gain more confidence in their bodies and the process of birth. It is my hope that regardless of views of how one's birth ought to be and with whom, that by reading this book, minds will be open and decisions will be made consciously and individually. There is no one right way and place to birth. However, there are truths that must be addressed. There are natural laws that are in motion. When these are fully understood and respected, there is peace and even joy.

I believe, as *Midwifery Today states,* that 'birth is as safe as life gets'. This is not a book for 'free birth-ers', 'home birth-ers, 'birth center birth-ers', or even 'hospital birth-ers'. This is a book for all birthing women and men who wish to participate fully in the process of the birth before them.

I would have one to understand that when we let *birth* proceed in an *unhindered way*, then the highest likelihood of safety, peace, joy and love will follow. This is the most essential beginning for life and will promote the ever important bond between mother, baby and father. This opportunity to greet life with peace, joy and love is the most essential step toward a successful life that one might ever have.

# Introduction

Over the last 20 years, I have been enthralled with and drawn to birth. I've seen enough lives impacted by this journey to know that the effect of childbirth on one's life is undeniably real. I've seen births deviate dramatically from the 'plan' that the parents had in mind and their deserved upset over this. I've seen births deviate dramatically from the 'plan' and parents come out with mixed emotions or even a peace and acceptance. And conversely, I've seen births go wonderfully ideal and according to the desires of the parents and these parents come out as if they had climbed a mountain; like they are new, more important and powerful individuals simply as a result of the transformation in them through their birth. It is this that I seek to share. It is this; this undeniable opportunity for individuals to embrace the journey of birth, with acceptance and empowerment coming out transformed and stronger. Stronger as a family, stronger as a mother, a father and stronger in everything that they do in life.

Much to the experience of my background as a Certified Childbirth Educator, through BirthWorks Inc., I have a strong belief that every woman will birth best where she feels the safest. It is the choice of each woman to choose that place and that care provider, if any at all. No woman should be pressured or condemned about her choice of where and how to birth. However, I strongly believe that if more women will face their fears surrounding birth and open their minds to learning, then these fears can be lessened, shifted and / or removed. It is often miss-information that causes the highest amount of fear. With the enormous amount of myths and fallacies in our society related to birth, it's no wonder that potentially dangerous and even threatening procedures and situations are accepted as the 'norm' or the protocol for a 'safe' birth. Through education and an open heart, we can dispel the ignorance that conforms us into what we feel is the only path to birth.

It is my hope that every woman on the journey through pregnancy and birth will be drawn to read this book. I pray then over their hearts that they can open up to their fears and reading these stories of growth and strength through birth, will come out with more peace and acceptance, if not eagerness, for the transformation that their births can bring. The stories represented in *Birth Unhindered* are varied in their location and use of birth attendants and circumstances. However, the common thread is that of unhindered birth. Birth that is allowed to happen spontaneously, without intervention. In the cases where there is intervention of any kind, the reader can contemplate for themselves how that affected the outcome and the impact on the birthing woman. There are conversely, stories with potentially harmful intervention to contrast the concept of unhindered birth. These stories are written by the women, from their perspective and only lightly edited for grammar.

No matter where or how a woman intends to birth, this book will be one of empowerment, helping her to achieve her desired results with birth. A father's fears also impact the birthing woman and child. For this reason, in addition to the desire to promote a strong bond with the baby, it is just as imperative that the father be given the opportunity to become empowered and engaged in the birth process. Because, when a birthing woman feels safe, there is peace and openness, and when there is peace and openness, babies come.

# Disclaimer

While I believe fully in the safety and purity of birth, I in no way, am stating that every woman should birth *without* assistance. I also am not stating that a woman should birth *with* assistance. The woman's instincts should always surpass the guidance and judgment of any outside source.

Choosing a certain place and way to give birth will, in no way, ensure safety. The claims and opinions found in *Birth Unhindered* are those of the author and the women who were generous enough to share their very real experiences. They are not construed as a guide in how to give birth.

Each woman/man should choose the setting, attendants and procedures that are right for their own situation.

Tara L. McGuire

Birth Works© Inc. Mission Statement:
Birth Works embodies the philosophy of developing a woman's self confidence, trust, and faith in her ability to give birth. It is the goal of our Childbirth Educator and Doula Certification Programs, and our childbirth classes, to promote safe and loving birth

experiences through education, introspection and confident action.

Vision Statement:

Birth Works© Inc. affirms that birth is an intensely felt and uniquely empowering transformation for women, babies, and families.

# My Journeys Through Birth by Tara:

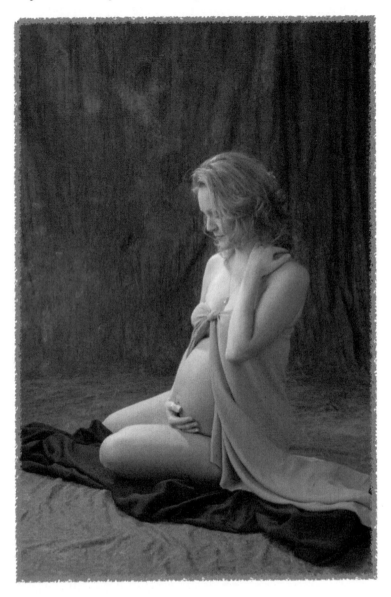

It seems that my journey through birth has been blessed from the start. And, when I say blessed, I mean that I started out ahead in the journey. I had loved ones who guided me and opened my mind.

It seems that I was spared the hard knocks, so to speak that are often experienced as a woman goes through her birthing years. This allowed me to have each birth be one that was a joy and helped to make me the woman that I am today.

I have been told that from a very young age, all I wanted was to grow up and be a mama. Even as young as 5 years old. It's interesting that I hear the same things from one of my girls. Although my journey began young, it's been full of highs and lows and everything in between. As I sit here and write, I am pregnant and due in two months to give birth for the fifth time. Only this time, it's not my baby........

My first experience began just four short months after graduating from high-school. My boyfriend and I had moved out of state to advance and pursue my modeling career, or so we thought. We had begun our wedding plans soon after summer had ended and expected to be married the next year on November 6th, 1993. As I had chosen a beautiful but expensive wedding gown that my father was about to purchase, I felt it was best that I confront a nagging concern. So, on November 6th of 1992, I took a pregnancy test. As I saw the two lines appear, I was in shock and scared. My boyfriend, Kent, was pounding on the bathroom door begging to be let in, as he heard me weep and two teenaged kids' worlds flipped upside down. We had a good deal of hugs and cries that day and quickly let go of the upset. We were both very family oriented and quickly became excited about our little one on the way. With some adjustments to our plans and direction in life at that time, we got married and began building our home.

It was easy for me to simply let go of the modeling path since being a mother had always been my deepest dream. My interest in pregnancy and mothering had been present even through high-school. Having had a friend give birth at 16 years of age, I thought I knew what I wanted; an epidural and an episiotomy. These are the ways to go, right? I had no idea that one person could completely alter the path before me. And yet, that's exactly what happened.

My Aunt Jean suggested that I meet her friend, a midwife. I had never even heard that word before. I was a young 18 year old and had lots of life to experience ahead of me. With much curiosity, I agreed to meet this woman. As Kent and I walked in to the home where the midwife worked, we were full of anticipation and ignorance. And then, out walked a pregnant angel. Her name was Charlotte and she stood just over five feet tall, with golden hair and a huge smile, only topped by her enormous belly. This was the midwife that we were to meet. I had no idea what this was all about, but I knew that I was supposed to be there and felt fearlessly led to follow this path.

I was shocked to learn that women birth outside of the hospital and that they even do so without drugs. This had me curious and eager to learn (since I quickly enlisted her services). I read with a voracious appetite, everything that I could get my hands on. I spent most of my pregnancy unemployed and totally engrossed in learning and preparing for the journey of birthing and mothering. This first pregnancy of mine was of enormous personal growth and blossoming as an individual.

*The Birth of Austin:*

Our EDD (estimated due date) for Austin was July 15th. I was so excited and eager for what birth is. I was up for the challenge! Labor began on the 24th of July with light contractions steadily but slowly progressing. Our parents came up from Oregon to be present for the birth. At this time, we shared a two bedroom apartment on the third floor with my brother and his wife and things were tight with all that company. Our midwife came at 3 AM on Monday the 26th and we all slept until around 7 AM. That morning, my midwife suggested nipple stimulation, and my ripe old age of 19 was not open to that! With heavily blushing cheeks, I said, 'no thanks'. We took walks and baths and not much was helping the progress. He was posterior, which means he is facing my belly rather than my back and this makes for a less effective labor.

Our midwife tried to break the bag of waters, but it wouldn't let go. After that, I took a shower and it broke on it's own! More walks and not much progress and I was getting very tired. Charlotte suggested I lay down and we found labor to be more effective. I needed a lot of counter-pressure on my back, but the rest and little bouts of sleep helped things along. At 5 PM, our midwives began nipple stimulation (without asking, but more informing) and an hour later, I was ready to push. The stronger contractions encouraged him to turn.

All of our family was outside the door, encouraging me and passing notes underneath and my mother was in the room for support. At 6:36 PM, Austin Lee was born with his dad catching him with assistance. He was 8 lb. 6 oz and 22 in long! I did it! Wow. We went through the normal clean up and settling in and let family come see and hold him, then we settled in for the night for the first time as parents.

Life as a mother suited me well. I doted on my little boy and adored him and my role. Keeping house and meeting my husband and son's needs was a joy. After a couple of years, I was aching again for another child. When Austin was a little over two, we tried to conceive again and were pregnant on the first try. I was thrilled and loved being pregnant again. Taking care of my son and resting when I needed seemed natural. Listening to classical music became a part of life then as I learned that it can increase the well being and IQ of the child. During this pregnancy, we found a home to purchase and left our apartment, moving into our first home just four weeks before my baby arrived. Boy, was I ready to have a new baby in my new home!

## The Birth of Jonah:

After Austin's birth, I was so excited to plan another home birth. I had, however, decided to interview all of the local midwives before I made a decision. I was eager to choose a lay midwife rather than a nurse midwife as I have learned that their approach to birth falls more in line with my beliefs. The decision was made and I was ready to get going on this pregnancy!

My due date was getting closer and I was getting anxious. On the 26th of September, I lost some of my mucus plug and I was instantly on a high. I just couldn't wait to meet my baby and honestly, I couldn't wait to be on the other side of having another empowering birth. That day, I saw Betty, my midwife, who said she would be on vacation from the 29th to the 6th of October and she really wanted me to be pregnant when she got back. I had already met her back up midwife and was sure God would let this baby come when it was right and I certainly wouldn't stand in the way.

On the 28th, I started loosening up in the bowels, had back aches and other general discomforts. The idea that the baby would be here soon was becoming more real. At 4:30 AM on Sunday the 29th, I started having some contractions. So, I got out of bed and started timing. They didn't amount to much.

That day, we went to church and then to my mom's house. All day long, I had diarrhea, lost mucus plug and had contractions that were irregular and infrequent. The idea that this will turn into the real thing is very hopeful.

Monday morning, the 30th, I have been having pretty regular contractions all night. Now I know it's not going to stop until I have my baby. I let Kent go to work and I couldn't wait to know when I will see my baby. My dad would be up, so I called him at 5:30 AM to let him know I'm in labor. My mom was next and she was coming right over. The excitement was thick in the air now. I had called the back up midwife, Lisa, the night before to let her know the baby would be here in a day or so. At 7 AM, my contractions were getting stronger, at 7-12 minutes apart. By now, I'm anxious to get working hard.

My mom arrived and we settled in and then took Austin for a walk to the playground. The walk all but stopped my contractions. At 2:40, my contractions are getting much stronger, but no closer. The pain is sharp near my cervix and I was intrigued as I hadn't felt that with my first.

At 3:30, Kent arrived and just as I had told my mom they would, my contractions got stronger and closer together. Mom kept Austin busy while Kent and I argued a little. We cleared the air and prayed together and settled into the flow of things. I thought a warm bath would help the sharp pain at my cervix. I knew my cervix was posterior at first, but checked it again and found it to have moved forward and I was dilated several centimeters.

Next, I soaked in a warm bath while Kent timed contractions. Stroking my lower abdomen seemed to help, but with the water on it, it seemed impossible to do, so Mom squirted oil on my belly, which felt great. It seemed that Kent was just now starting to realize what kind of pain that I was really in. And yet, I was still cherishing the process. I knew I was OK.

Mom and Austin walked into the bathroom at this point with snacks. Austin carried a tray of cheese, crackers, and chocolate covered Oreos. My mom had root-beer in our champagne glasses. Along with the candle light, it made a very calm and sweet setting.

After the bath, I dressed and we decided to call Lisa to come. She wasn't at home, so we paged her. The contractions were becoming much stronger and the stroking no longer helped. I had to hold onto someone. Most of the time it was Kent. Just holding him made it more bearable. I was having a hard time breathing. I felt like I was hyperventilating. So, I tried using some patterned breath that I had learned and it seemed to help slow down the intake. It was hard for me to believe, but the pain was stronger than with my first, however, I still wasn't discouraged. I had been so eager for this.

My mom got Austin to bed and put on some relaxing music. I felt like I could really do it now. I had moved out into the living room, sitting in a rocker with my mother and Kent by my side. 7 PM and still no answer from the midwife. So, we called her husband who also couldn't reach her or her assistant (we later found out that there was a problem with the local tower that transmits the pages). During this time, my mother and Kent rubbed me during contractions. Always needing my back rubbed and any other touch was helpful. During this time, we were joking about birthing without a midwife. Kent didn't like that at all! Now we were starting to worry. Contractions are getting very strong at 4-5 minutes apart.

At 8:15, we get the phone book out. Having interviewed the midwives earlier in the year, I knew this was a better option than going into the hospital. We finally reached Carol, who lived in another near-by city, but her supplies were in yet another near-by city. It would be a bit of time. We were relieved but wondered if she would make it. It was 8:45 PM and the thought of going to the hospital was not even remotely present.

I hadn't gone to the bathroom the whole time we were waiting for confirmation that someone was coming. So, up mom and I go while Kent was on the phone giving Carol directions. Wow, the contractions I had on the toilet were incredible. All I could do was hold on to my mom and try my best to breathe. Carol gave orders for me to go lay down and get off the pot. No Kidding! 'It's kind of hard to move during that kind of pain', I thought.

So, into the bedroom we go. I wasn't on the bed long when I realized that I was in transition, or the last phase of dilation. It was such a struggle to breathe through the contractions. Kent was a big help with that. Mom rubbed my leg and reminded me to relax my arms and shoulders. Mom asked if everything was ready, like hot compresses. So, I told them to fill the crock-pot with hot water and put it in the bathroom. The air was thick with anticipation and a little fear. Although, the soft candle light and the soothing music helped.

Soon, I was feeling an urge to push and remember saying that I hoped that was an urge for a bowel movement even though I

21

knew otherwise. From then on, I kept asking Kent when Carol would arrive. At about 9:15, my body started pushing the baby out. I tried panting and blowing to stop, but there was no stopping this powerful reflex. I've never felt so out of control of my body. Knowing that I wanted to wait for the midwife, but unable to stop my body. Kent had a hard time understanding that the pushing was out of my control and kept instructing me to stop. When I felt the head move down, I felt a warm mess between my legs and told them to take my panties off. Kent's eyes got as big as saucers and said, 'Now I AM scared'. This must have been the point that he dialed 911.

Still laying on my side, mom cleaned me up and I reached in to see where the head was. We had about two inches. On the next contraction, mom told Kent to get the compresses. She could see the head. Mom and I were doing our best to calm Kent and myself as well.

I realized that I needed to roll over and mom worked on my perineum helping it to not tear with hot compresses and support. The head was born quickly and he was squawking immediately. With the next push, I joined in. Kent helped work the shoulders out while mom made sure his airway was clear. The baby was still half in and half out and kicking me on the inside. I told them to pull it out. He was laid on my belly and covered with a blue pad. his color was perfect and he was perfect. Another son. We were all so relieved.

During all of this action on the bed, Kent was on the phone, following the instructions of the 911 tech and they were always a step behind and pointless. I found it irritating, but know he was just trying to do his best and keep us safe. I now find it interesting to type this up in detail and see how afraid we were to not have a professional there.

Kent, still frantic, was terrified that I had torn. We assured him that I was fine and encouraged him to look at the baby. The paramedics arrived about 2 minutes later and stood in my room like wall hangings. About a minute or two later, Carol arrived. After the men got a little info, they left. Carol was such a welcomed sight. She took care of the placenta and all the other necessary procedures.

Jonah Michael weighed 7 lbs 6 oz and was 21 inches long. What a beautiful experience! Sleepy little Austin was brought in, but wasn't interested. Kent then cut the cord. We cleaned up and I dressed Jonah with mom's help and he nursed well. I didn't even have the slightest abrasion. How remarkable! Kent and I lay with our son, just in shock that we did this on our own. How *AMAZING!* How empowering. It was beautiful.

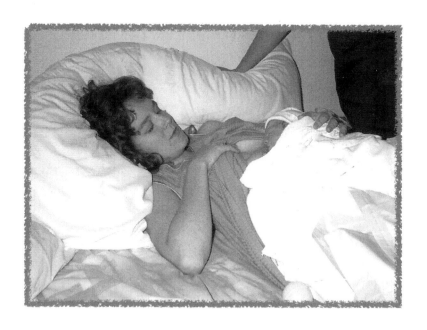

*My Interim of Infertility and Loss:*

Once Jonah was a little over a year, my heart led me to learn about becoming a certified childbirth educator. This process was fun for me as it took me into deeper learning and exploration. I became certified through Birth Works© Inc. and started teaching about a year and a half after his birth. I loved working with birthing couples and helping them become educated and make informed decisions about birth. Through this, I really knew that I was impacting their future and the futures of the babies born more peacefully and gently into the world.

It wasn't long and I was aching for a baby again and namely; a girl! I had dreamed of having a little girl for as long as I could remember and we began trying. Month after month, I didn't conceive and each month that I had a period broke my heart and weakened my confidence in my body. I began seeing doctors for symptoms that I was having; some related to fertility and some not. It was what seemed like forever before I became pregnant and we were elated. This elation turned into disbelief as I began to spot, bleed and then miscarry at 9 weeks. I was broken, but not surprised as my investigation had shown that I was conceiving regularly, but not carrying. Women actually have pregnancy loss much more than they realize.

We continued working on conceiving and continued to have no results. I began to suffer more and more ill health and saw several different doctors. Depression set in and it was the toughest point of my life so far. This time, it took twice as long to conceive again and when I did, we were excited, but afraid to get our hopes up. As things progressed, we gained hope and at 11 weeks, I began spotting. I immediately went to the DR for an ultrasound because my heart and mind just could not wait like before. It was found that the baby was gone and there was no hope. I was offered a D&C and gladly accepted. I just needed to be over it. I wasn't strong enough at that point to wait out a spontaneous miscarriage. The depression grew worse and life grew darker as I continued to teach my birthing classes and worked with birthing couples. I continued to see doctors and my last visit was shocking.

I can remember, in vivid detail, the smell of the office, the look of the room and the feel of the chair that I sat on when the DR told me that I was in the early stages of Lupus. He proceeded to tell me what to expect ahead of me. At that point, I drew inward. It was like a fog. Like someone was playing a movie in front of me that I wasn't watching. By the time that he was done speaking, an internal fire was ablaze. I was infuriated that I was there. I was infuriated that he was telling me this. I was infuriated that I let myself get to this point of losing faith and trust in my body. I was infuriated that I had lost the deep belief that our minds and spirits create the body that we live in. I said nothing, thanking him calmly and left. I never went back. Something inside of me had changed.

At this point, I poured myself into learning about herbs, and health and nutrition. I had this deep belief that if we put our bodies in the right environment and give it the right elements, they can heal themselves. During this time, I also checked into our insurance and wanted to see if I would be covered for seeing a fertility specialist. I felt that if I could find out what was off' in my body, then I could learn how to support and balance that issue. Our insurance would provide coverage for the diagnosis, but not the treatment and we proceeded to begin testing.

This was a time of empowerment for me. Months of learning, and employing nutritional changes and looking within myself to find out what my fears really were. I meditated and found a scripture in the Bible that gave me enormous strength. 'Everything you ask for in prayer will be yours if you only have faith'. Mark 11:24. I began meditating on my good health and fertility. It was at this time that Kent and I were given a trip to Hawaii through his employer. I decided that this trip would be when I would conceive and that this would be a wonderful and strong pregnancy and that it would be a girl. I worked hard in building this belief. The timing in my cycle was perfect and my spirit was strong. I was claiming the results that I desired! After two years, the pain could end.

A couple of weeks after we returned from Hawaii, I was facing the deadline and my faith wavered. I was afraid to be let down after two years of trying and losing babies. But, I simply spent more time praying and reading and believing. When I took that pregnancy test and two lines appeared, I was overjoyed and affirmed! Kent shared my joy, but not having been going through this inner struggle for personal growth, he was more cautious about having hope, much less faith.

Because we had been going through the fertility clinic to find a diagnosis, they were the ones watching me early on. They set an appointment for an ultrasound at 8 weeks and I felt indignant to have that intrusion. I knew that she was there and that she was perfect. I was on cloud 9. And then, around the 9th week, I began spotting. My heart sank, but somewhere in me, I knew things were OK and I prayed. Hard. I spoke with the women in my life and many had spotting during healthy pregnancies. So, the spotting stopped and we drudged on.

This pregnancy was tough on me physically and I was very sick with morning sickness. I had also been with Jonah, but didn't know to explore options for relief. My midwife this time was Carol. She gave me some relief that I swear by. The ancient wisdom and learning of a midwife is admirable. Once things lightened up and I felt better, I cherished my growing belly and blossoming breasts. I just knew that I was as beautiful and wonderful as I would ever be.

*The Birth of Faith:*

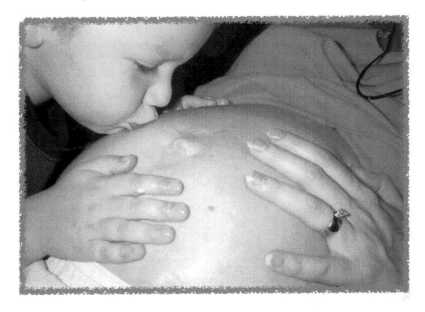

We had an EDD of October 31st with this baby. Halloween. Interesting for a family that doesn't celebrate. However, I had a feeling that we wouldn't go that long. Friday the 6th, at night time, I was cramping with some back ache and loose stools. I was very PMSy. Like my hormones had shifted. All night long I was crampy. Saturday the 7th, we went to the coast and I had regular, light contractions with loose stools. However, they quit at night time. I knew my body was getting ready, but I was so eager to meet my little girl! On Sunday the 8th, I had more regular and stronger contractions with a strong nesting instinct. So, I am working on letting this come at it's own pace......*Trust.*

Monday the 9th, I had light and irregular contractions and my midwife found me to be 3 cm dilated, 90% effaced and losing mucus plug. We're starting to really get excited! Tuesday the 10th, more of the same, but feeling discouraged as contractions have lessened and I am eager. I took mineral oil, cohosh, and did breast stimulation. Only light contractions and I had to re-evaluate and remind myself that babies come when they are ready.

Wednesday the 11th, we went to a doctor visit for my son to get some stitches removed and I knew that I didn't need any more stress that day! We went out for Mexican food and it was fantastic. I had regular contractions and thought I might as well help them by taking castor oil. OUCH! So much for relaxing and letting things happen on their own, right? I wasn't sure why for almost a week, my body was acting like it was going into labor, but wouldn't. I didn't have that before. It's funny how we expect what we are familiar with. I had a good labor pattern as a result of all of this and my family came over.

Thursday the 12th, now 4 cm and 80% effaced? The head is lower, though. Contractions stopped. Everyone went home and I again had to re-evaluate the process. I wouldn't be pregnant forever, right? She knows when it's time, right? Just relax and enjoy the last bit of pregnancy. But, I am so eager to meet my baby! For the next two weeks, I experienced this pre-labor. I call it pre-labor because it does good things to prepare the body for birth. This was a very tough time as I was uncomfortable almost the whole time with contractions and cramping. Tuesday morning the 24th, my midwife and I decided to simply stretch the cervix. She also gave me a homeopathic to induce labor. At this point, I was already 5 cm and effaced completely. Not even in 'real' labor. I was baffled and it was testing my strength and patience after 2 1/2 weeks.

Contractions began again around 11 AM and were my typical sporadic, irregular contractions. They were close together (2-3 min) and we were told they would spread out and get stronger. We spent the day waiting for this and living life as usual. I felt no different than I had for the past couple of weeks. After dinner at 5 PM, I was lighting candles and felt one of these little contractions come on and out of frustration, thought, 'what the heck, I'll squat and see what happens'. During that little contraction, I felt a double snap and water went everywhere. I was in shock and it took a moment to realize that my water broke. I hollered for someone to bring me a towel. I then moved into the bathroom to remove my drenched clothes and clean up. Directly after, I went to my bed and lay on my side to hopefully see what was going to happen. We called Carol and she was promptly on her way. This time, she knew a shorter path.

Meanwhile, mom and Kent were getting things ready. The contractions were immediately intense. THIS is labor. I lay on the bed praying Carol and my friend Michelle, would make it and that I would have time to get into the birth tub. My next thought was my urgent need to have a bowel movement but knowing that if I got up and sat on the toilet, I would have a baby right then and there. I was unwilling to go. We were waiting for Carol and the tub. I was amazed at the intensity of the labor.

Carol arrived and began getting supplies ready. I knew then that I couldn't go to the bathroom because I was paralyzed by the intensity and because the baby would pop out. I kept asking if the tub was ready and was told that it was too hot. I remember being angry at this and demanded hot compresses. I then felt the baby coming and said so. Carol and my mom came in. The baby and the contents of my bowels moved down. UGH and uck. I was then glad to have the midwife there. After this, I was given the pleasure of hot compresses on my perineum and it felt like such relief as the baby crowned.

My mother brought the boys in a couple of contractions later, her head popped out just as my mother in law came in the front door. My noises scared Jonah and he began crying. Brenda (mother in law), came in and another contraction came then the baby's shoulder started coming. I watched as I pushed the baby out. The baby was then laid on my tummy and covered with the most near-by item, which happened to be a dishtowel. We were admiring the baby and Kent was asking what sex the baby was. I was confused for a bit as I *knew* I was having a girl. I then lifted the towel and saw. Everyone asked with excitement and I said, 'It's my Faith, of course'. The joy and excitement was electric, but I was just filled with peace. Calm after a 30 minute labor.

Her brothers came in and were enjoying looking her over. My friend Michelle then arrived and began videoing. A few minutes later I was covered with a towel and my father in law came in to see us. Shortly after, my parents came in and after everyone went out, we got into the birth tub. Just Faith and I with candles burning and beautifully soothing Celtic music playing. It was just what we needed after an intense birth. How amazing that I had signs of labor and my body was 'trying' to go into labor for weeks and then this overwhelmingly fast labor and birth. It was such a shock.

Faith latched on right away and nursed the whole time we were in the tub. She was so beautiful and tiny. We got out of the tub and went to our now cleaned bed. People were coming and going, saying their congrats and peeking at my beautiful babe nursing at my breast. Big brothers spent most of the next hours as close and as chatty as can be. After all was settled and everyone left, mom, dad and Faith snuggled in for the night. What a journey that I had been on for three years. She lay on my left shoulder and I stared at her literally all night long. Kent woke in the morning and found me still gazing at her. He asked, 'did you get any sleep?', to which I peacefully smiled and shook my head no. Her first name is

Faith, her middle name is Manalani, which is Hawaiian for 'heavenly power'. 8 lbs and 20 in. October 24th, 2000, I am a new woman.

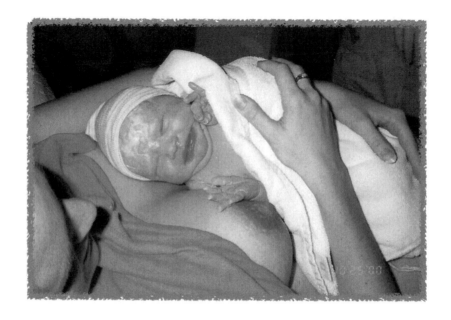

*Interim of Transition:*

Life with another baby was blissful even though she was colicky and the only way to bring the most relief was for me to quit eating dairy and wheat. Her intolerance of these made her quite uncomfortable. It was simple, and natural for me to sleep with her, to carry her most of the time and I never had an inclination to pump so that she could take a bottle and be away from me. Faith was a real healing for me and I delighted in her. A little over a year after her birth, some of the previous symptoms that I had been experiencing began to return and I just didn't feel that same level of health that I knew was possible. It was when she was one and a half that I found a health and wellness company that gave me the highest level of health that I have ever experienced. During these years, my marriage had been struggling. We were having a harder and harder time as we continued to grow up and into different people.

Four months after getting myself onto these wellness products, I missed a period. This was devastating and confusing. I had worked so hard and tried so long to have Faith and now I was content, wanting no more children. Things were already tough at home and I really didn't know how having another baby was going to change things. Sure enough, I was pregnant. This was tough for me to accept and I cried a lot. It seemed so odd that I had such a tough journey and then just getting my body into a healthy state, I was pregnant while trying to avoid it. In a similar way, I again felt very out of control.

I knew one thing for sure; if I was going to have another baby, it was going to be my way, with no influence from others or what I thought I was 'supposed' to do. I knew that I wanted to let go of 'control' in this pregnancy. To totally open up to the process I needed to not 'know' everything. I needed to just simply experience. I had deepened my trust in the process of pregnancy and birth and it was time for me to live fully in that. In a way, my displeasure of having another baby was a catalyst for the most empowering experience of my life. I chose to go completely unassisted for the journey. I took no pregnancy test. I didn't enlist a midwife. I just simply let the natural process unfold before me. My prenatal care was in my hands and consisted of my eating well, doing yoga and praying. I wrote and I was guided by my intuition. It seemed that allowing myself to have my baby my way was my comfort and consolation for having another child that I didn't plan on.

*The Birth of Grace:*

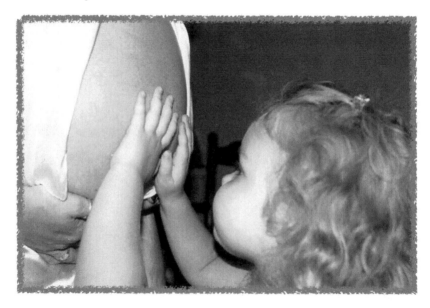

It's July, 2003 and my body is round and full of baby. I am feeling ready to meet this little one. I've begun my pre-labor workout and we are wondering when the day will be. We have had a few hopeful days that only turn into restful nights and mornings of empty arms. I go back and forth in my mind if I should 'help' things along by encouraging labor, or wait and trust that God is in control. Babies know when to be born. After two and a half weeks of having contractions and fighting and wanting to be in control, I have surrendered to the process.

It is the night of the 15th and I am having contractions that I am sleeping through. As morning comes, it is 3:30 AM and I can no longer sleep through them as my back is hurting very much. 4 AM and I get up and go out onto the couch to see what happens. Contractions keep coming and feel like real labor. I am wondering and hopeful that today is the day! Could it be that I will be holding my babe this very day? I wake Kent and tell him we need to begin filling the birth tub. This takes several hours. Resting on the couch some more, contractions become stronger and I am beginning to believe that this is it. I get out my PalmMag (a magnetic device) for my back that is hurting so much. This takes care of my back discomfort and leaves only the sensation of the contractions. 5:30 AM and I am sure this is it!!! So, I get on the computer to send emails.

I have been craving doughnuts all morning and when Kent gets up to finish the tub at 7 AM, I ask him to go get some. So, as he realizes he is not going into work, off he goes to get me a doughnut. To make sure that I will have energy, I drink a protein drink mixed with barley grass. I then call my friend and mother to let them know that I am in labor. Now my two sons and daughter are up and very excited that today is the day! Contractions take my focus at this point as they are painful. No one is timing. No one is measuring. It is all so normal and relaxed. The whole pregnancy has been like that and helped me fall in love with my babe.

Kent arrives with doughnuts and we work to corral the children and make order of our nest. It's around 8 AM now and I am very eager to get in the tub and relax. All morning I have had thoughts of this baby coming too quickly and I have sensed myself holding back for fear of this. But, as we get more things in place, I begin to see that it is all going according to my vision. I keep thinking how wonderful it is to be in labor and have 'normal' contractions and normal breaks in between. My last birth was so fast that it was like being ran over by a train. Now I am climbing into the birth tub and I just melt. My tension is gone and all we are waiting for is my friend to come. I keep thinking how badly the sensations hurt and keep focused on staying relaxed and welcoming. At this point, I have to have my husband touching me to keep me breathing steady and relaxed. I am beginning to over heat but don't look forward to the more intense labor that will come when I leave the water.

Just then I hear my friend come through the door and I know we can get serious.

Around 9 AM now and I am getting out of the tub. As I empty my bladder, I am thankful I don't have to stay there long and endure the constant contractions that are inevitable. I want to take time and enjoy my labor dance. We've spread a shower curtain and sheet in the living room and this is where I labor in the company of Kent and Brandi for an hour or so. As a wave builds in me, I find a forward leaning position and let Kent know to touch me. Occasionally, I have Brandi press her thumb into the middle of my palm and rub. As my back is hurting worse, I have Kent roll a magnetic massager around my sacrum during contractions. This brings great relief.

I have lost all sense of time and space and am riding purely on sensation. Now I know I must get back into the water. A quick empty of the bladder and I slide into the tub. What joy! Upon checking, I seem to be nearly completely dilated and the waters are still intact. Although I keep waiting for the sensations to come back to back, they don't. And during them, I am thinking how badly they hurt. Inside myself, I want to run and escape. I feel a panic and must focus to breathe slowly and not hyperventilate. I tell myself, 'I can do this.' 'I was created to do this.' Each break, I find it amazing that I remain calm, polite and even cheerful at times.

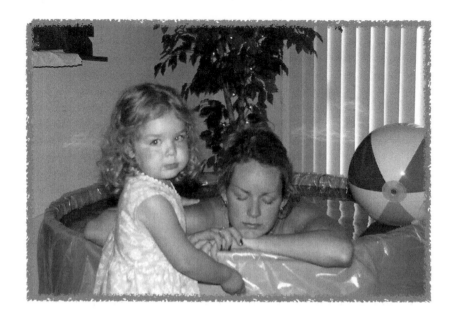

As the contractions don't seem to be moving the baby and the bag of waters, I assume a squat which is pleasantly easy in the water. Now I feel a catch in my throat as I work with the sensations. So, I try pushing gently and find the pain to lessen. I like that and go with it. Now I feel the baby moving down and am beginning to experience the involuntary pushing of my body; the primal power within that brings our babies out. Kent and Brandi are working cameras now and I lean back and get against the back of the tub so that I can see and catch my babe. As the next rush sweeps over me, I feel my body being split apart. I am overwhelmed as I passively surrender to my body as it births. I expect the head to crown, but it keeps coming and I reach to support the skin that is not responding so quickly. The baby's head comes and we call for the children just as the bag of waters bursts, propelling baby into mine and dad's hands. Surprised by the speed, we pull her to my chest. HER?! I was expecting a boy! Sure enough, it is a girl. The children are all so thrilled but none as much as our two year old who just got a real live baby doll!

Grace Anna is born at 11:42 AM on July 16th, 2003. We enjoy an hour or so in the tub together nursing and bonding. We then manage to get out and go to the bedroom to wait for the placenta. After a bit, we tie and cut the cord. This takes some fussing as we have never tied the cord ourselves.

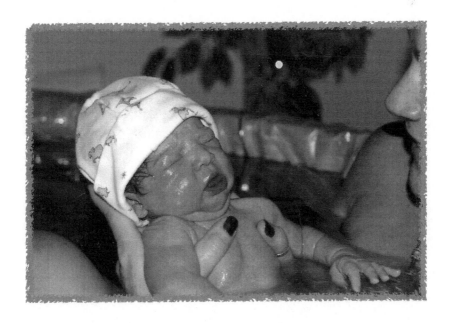

Still no placenta and Brandi suggests that I get back into the tub where it will be much more comfortable to empty my bladder and wait for the placenta. It is very comfortable in the water, but still no placenta and I am eager to get on with things. I elevate myself and get our little Grace back in with me to nurse.

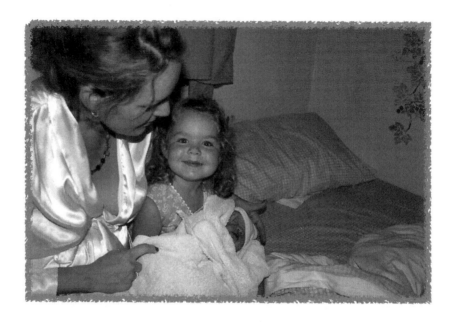

Still nothing, so I drink some very strong red raspberry leaf tea and feel a strong contraction. I quickly am handing (more like throwing), Grace over due to the pain. I bear down and out comes the placenta, followed by that enormous sense of relief only a birthing woman knows. I am done and it feels so incredible. Now I climb out and go take a quick shower. This is where we climb into bed as a new family of six. Life is good. God is good and so full of Grace! Now, I have no doubt that there isn't anything in life that I cannot do. This is what every woman deserves.

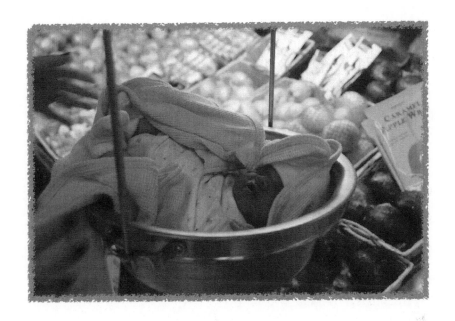

The next day, we took Grace to the grocery store and weighed her in the produce scale. She weighed 7 lbs even. We were so proud of our journey, but none more than me. I trusted. I accepted my fears. I listened to my intuition and it was a blessed event. *I'll never be the same.*

My Journey Through Surrogacy:

A few years after the birth of Grace, my husband and I divorced. Now faced with being a single, home-schooling mom of four, life was interesting, to say the least. It was as if I had this overwhelming excitement about being able to be and do anything that I wished. I became a Yoga instructor. I played with real estate, and remodeled and flipped a piece of real-estate and made a profit. Toward the end of 2008, I was considering what I wanted to do with the rest of my life and the fact that I would be turning 35 the next year seemed to weigh heavily on me. Not in a bad way, but more of a mile marker. I recalled the past desire to be a surrogate for an infertile couple and the more I considered this, the more I wanted to do it. And, against my boy-friend's advice, I stepped out and pursued a match. It was amazing to me that it only took one profile on a website and I was flooded with inquiries. After only a couple of weeks, I had found the couple that I knew in my heart I was intended to be matched with.

This couple lived in Australia but were from Israel. It seemed that our connection was instant and strong and I was as excited as could be to be looking toward the empowering experience of bringing a child into the world and the added benefit of not having to raise that child! It took a few months of setting the contract and putting together the team of professionals that would make this happen, but finally, at the end of March, I flew to La Jolla and met the intended mother for the first time. On April 2nd, I was laid on a table and with her hand in mine, the doctor inserted two 5 day old beings into my uterus. I'll never forget how after my three days of bed rest, we said goodbye, tears in her eyes for leaving her little ones' futures so far out of her control.

The days that I had to wait to see if the embryos implanted were long, but I was sure that I would end up pregnant and I did. The parents were overjoyed when I shared the good news. This surrogacy required daily shots of hormones and pills to support the pregnancy and these medications made me feel sick. I experienced a level of sickness unimaginable and I began regretting my decision. Operating as a single mom of four and home-schooling, while teaching yoga and being severely sick was more than I could handle. And yet, I was there. The normal approaches to managing this didn't make much impact this time, but thankfully the pregnancy progressed healthily.

As the parents wished for a hospital birth, I was placed under the care of an MD for the first time ever for prenatal care. Actually, it was a group of MDs. The contrast in care from a midwife to a doctor was staggering to me. I was thankful that I was experienced and educated as the way I was handled was quite inadequate, in my opinion. My body went through some signs of being overwhelmed by the level of my activity and the physical strain on me. So, at the beginning of the third trimester, I was put on work leave and asked to stop doing yoga all together. The parents were quite nervous and concerned for their child and I honored their request.

The last trimester was uncomfortable for me as my body began feeling very unnatural from the lack of yoga and typical pregnancy symptoms seemed huge. At 35 weeks, I began my familiar pre-

45

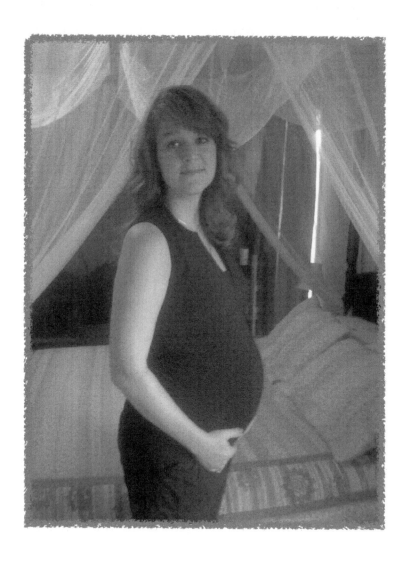

labor pattern. With the parents so far away in Australia and not intending to arrive until 38 weeks, this created much stress. However, we did make it. The weeks of pre-labor were not what they had been with my last in that I was not relaxed and accepting. I was annoyed and miserable. I was frustrated and somewhat regretful. By the end, I had almost no connection to the baby that I carried although I was just as careful in caring for myself and her. I just was ready to be done.

Because of my birth history, I informed the parents that their baby could come quite fast since I was having so much pre-labor. The MDs offered to just bring me in and induce me, of course because that is the typical solution to any problem, it seems. I began missing my appointments so that I didn't have to deal with their pressure. I told the parents that they should meet my midwife and they agreed. We had a lovely dinner with the midwife and her husband and the parents were able to ask a lot of questions and feel re-assured by the professionalism and care that the midwife could offer. She would be there no matter whether we could make it to the hospital or not.

On December 6th, my body was being a bit more convincing that the birth would be soon and now that the parents were in town, I was more than ready. As Carol had intended to come by the next day to check on me, I told her that night how I was feeling and she might want to call me first thing in the morning. When Carol called, I told her that I thought I was leaking fluid and was having contractions. So, she decided to come right over.

When Carol checked me, she found me to be maybe half way dilated and just then my water gushed everywhere. Once we cleaned up, contractions changed and intensified. I went to the toilet and began to be overwhelmed with labor. Immediately, I went to my tub and worked with my man on coping with the more intense labor than I had ever experienced. The midwife was noticing decelerations in the baby's heart rate in certain positions and it seemed that the only position that the baby favored did not feel good at all to me. The pain was so intense that I was hyperventilating and vomiting until the point that I was dry-heaving. I felt as if all the pain in the world were being born in my sacrum. This might be a good time to point out that I broke my tailbone a few years prior.

I began pushing and heard the phone ringing. The parents were calling to check on me, but I could not let Carol or Don leave my side. Carol wanted to keep a close listen to the baby and I had to have Don's touch. I was crying, complaining and even to my surprise, wishing for drugs. Why was I going through this and not going to be having a baby for me? It seemed to be too much. Carol took a quick minute to call the parents and tell them to come because it was too late to move me.

I was pushing and nothing was happening. Carol checked me and found that my cervix was now posterior and pushing would not do any good until it moved forward. She offered to hold the forward lip of the cervix down while I pushed a time or two and I eagerly accepted anything that would help. Because of the heart decels, we all felt compelled to get the baby out as soon as possible. Sure enough, with a couple of pushes, the baby's head made it through the cervix just as the parents came in the room.

The intensity of the pain seemed to be more than I could bare and yet the urge to push was almost non-existent. But my desire to get this baby born was *Big*. I was pushing and screaming at the top of my lungs as she came through what is called 'military style', with her head and neck straight, chin not tucked. The whole time I was screaming, in between breaths, I was apologizing to the mother that I was being noisy. Her and I had discussed this topic early in the pregnancy as she wasn't sure that she could be present for the birth largely due to the noise she expected me to make. I re-assured her that I do not make much noise at all when birthing. Well, nothing about this pregnancy seemed the same and it was so with the birth as well.

This little girl was laid on my belly, all thick with vernix and born at 38 weeks. She was perfect and all I could think about was how glad I was that the pain stopped. I was almost giddy. Just chatting and chatting. With my man, my midwife and this eager couple standing in the bathroom, we waited for the cord to finish pulsing before it was cut. I then handed her over to her dad and tears filled everyone's eyes as the parents held their little girl for the first time ever. Mikayla was 7 lbs, 2 oz and 19 inches long.

Everyone was ushered out soon after when we realized my bleeding was heavy. We shut the door so not to distress anyone and Carol gave me a shot of pitocin to stop the bleeding. It seemed that my placenta was again not eager to come out and my uterus was being lazy due to the fact that there was not a baby nursing to help. We were massaging it and I was still filling the tub with blood. As I was feeling light headed, Carol wanted to get me out and lay me down in bed. The tub was drained and when it was, we could see many huge blood clots in the bottom of the tub. I birthed the placenta, to my overwhelming relief and when I stood, I was shocked by the look of my feet. Feeling dazed and whoozy, I thought that they looked like I was dead. My boyfriend shared that I looked like a corpse as I had lost so much blood.

Once placed on my bed, I was able to eat and watch the midwife examine this new baby and show her parents how to care for her. This was a time of newness and excitement and shortly after, I nursed her. For five days, this new family stayed in my home and I nursed the baby that I carried. At that point, they moved out into a near by condo and came each day for several hours of visiting and nursing. I pumped and supplied the milk during this time also. At four weeks, we said good bye and they returned home. The time nursing was so sweet and special, creating a strong bond between this little baby and me. It was a time of healing and attachment that I hadn't intended on. At four weeks, the new family left for home and it was the second most difficult experience of my life. I've carried a blog and written a book about my surrogacy experience, to be published in 2011. The blog is tarasurrogacy.blogspot.com.

I've spent much time reflecting on why this pregnancy and birth were so difficult for me and besides the obvious influence of the medications, I feel it was due to the emotional and psychological dynamics involved. I was unable to process the emotions involved with this pregnancy due to the fear of attachment and loss. On the other side of the whole experience, I am now six weeks postpartum and still pumping. I will ship the milk that I have pumped in one more week so that my surrogate baby will have more of my milk.

It seems strange that my reproductive years are being wrapped up by such a unique and challenging experience, and yet, I accept it. I had my beautiful and perfect births. This one was what it needed to be. I also believe that because of the traumatic birth, I am a different person. I am more laid back and accepting of life and circumstance. It taught me to surrender to circumstance that I would not choose and this is a healthy skill.

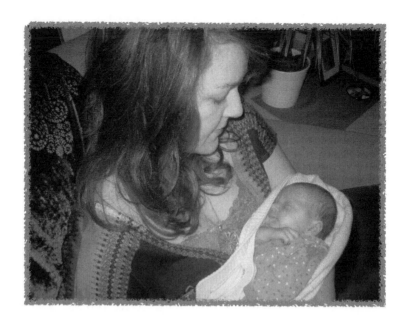

Now that I have had five experiences of birth, I feel I really am very balanced as a person. I know how to be strong when needed. I can be giving and yielding. I can be open and tender and I believe in my ability to take whatever comes my way and make it an experience to remember.

# Prenatal Care

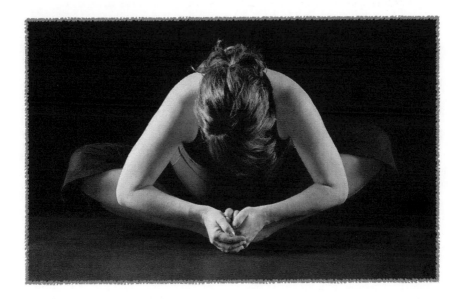

It's interesting how our society views health and the medical system. However, you would be hard pressed to deny that it's evolving. This change has been deeply needed, but it's still fraught with deceptions. Take the prenatal care that most women receive from an OB, for example. Everything that you are subjected to is to look for disease or disorder. It is as if we know something will go wrong and we are looking for it. Is this good for every woman to be subjected to? I'm not altogether sure.

The psychological impact on a pregnant woman of being 'guilty' until proven 'innocent' is subtle, but powerful on a society as a whole. I am very grateful that we do live in a time where, in most countries, a mother and baby can receive wonderful medical intervention when truly necessary and in the USA, there is no doubt that our medical system is quite skilled in the treatment of disease. Enter here the distinction. OBs and MDs are in the business of disease management. They are skilled professionals in the field of looking out for, detecting and labeling deviations from the normal process of birthing.

But what of health? What of the normal, physiological process of pro-creation? It is not a state of disease, but a completely natural and normal part of the life cycle. So, why are the experts in disease leading the 'care' of the normal processes of life? I will be the first to say that there is a huge schism between doctors and midwives. These breeches in what ought to be cohesive partnering in a mutual field are often fraught with egos, insecurities, and unbalanced and biased judgments. It is my hope that we will one day be able to see that the midwife is in a respectable collaboration with the OBs and MDs and that they can see that their field is the same, but their focus is quite different. They really ought to be complimentary. However, that would mean that there are many more midwives and much fewer doctors attending births.

There are great doctors and there are doctors who cause harm. There are great midwives and there are midwives who cause harm. However, when evaluating a system, one must be willing to make judgments and generalizations in order to see the bigger picture. So, for the sake of seeing just that, let me make these generalizations in order to make my points.

If doctors are the experts in disease and midwives are the experts in facilitating a normal physiologic outcome of childbirth, what is the difference in the the prenatal care administered by each? There is this huge and intentional deception that disease management *IS* prenatal care. I can tell you that my having had three pregnancies overseen by a midwife, one managed solely by me and the last managed by a group of physicians, what truly mattered in the end was the 'care' that I administered myself! Each woman should guard her own prenatal care as her own responsibility. A midwife will spend time counseling a woman on how to manage such things and an OB will talk for two minutes a visit about such things (if you are lucky) and give you a nicely printed hand out to take home. The focus is for the DR at each visit to make sure that you have had your appropriate screenings and tests and then to 'sell' you on the next. Each visit is heavy with what risks you are either currently facing or which risks are coming up.

Please hear me when I say, prenatal care is the simple act of nurturing yourself and your baby, body, mind and spirit! There is nothing complicated about it. It is not the screening for disease and deviations from normal. If you care to participate in that, you will choose a professional to do so. Here, I will outline the most essential components in good prenatal care. I simply outline because there are many books out there that go over these things in great detail.

•Walk 3-5 times a week. Get out doors and get your body moving and heart rate up. This is a mood lifter and good fitness. The cardio effect purifies the blood.

•Do yoga. I can't get away from this one. As a yoga teacher, I have found that the benefit is invaluable in reducing body discomforts due to tension and weakness. By practicing yoga, you will increase the flow of Chi in the body, enhancing yours and your baby's overall health. The way that yoga strengthens the body awareness spills over into benefit for labor, birth and mothering.

• Drink Lots of pure, clean and living water. There are many differences in water quality. Take the time to learn and choose a water purification system that makes sense to you. It is easy to get dehydrated while pregnant and this can bring on fatigue, discomforts and contractions. The amnionic fluid is continually recycled and is completely new every ten hours!

•Eat living food and often. Eating light and frequently will ensure that you are keeping a steady supply of energy flowing through for both you and your baby. Listen to how you feel when you eat a food. If you feel good and energized, then it is good for you. If you don't, then don't eat it. Your body's wisdom is best and often during pregnancy, a woman cannot tolerate certain things. Most often, the offender is animal product. You may find yourself able only to eat what grows from the ground. The more your food does not come from wrappers, the better. Protein seems to be the most essential and also the most un-met component while pregnant. Focus on eating a good protein source every time you eat.

•Supplement. This is a BIG topic, but with the state of soil depletion in the USA and our absolute inability to take in the ideal balance of nutrients from our food, it is a good idea to find a source for these missing nutrients. Admittedly, some individuals find that they are able to go through life with good health without the aid of supplementation. But that is the exception and not the rule. There is a way to get organic, whole food concentrates that are both safe and effective at replacing missing nutrients in your diet. Pregnancy is no time to be neglectful in this area.

•Rest every day. Even if you are not a napper, take time out each day to recline and rest. Some women couldn't avoid this even if they wanted to and find that they practically drop each day for a nap. Your body is working hard to grow another being and needs rest to do a good job of it.

•Laugh and cry. Allow yourself to have fun and to also feel the normal emotions that seem to be so close to the surface during pregnancy. You may find that you cry at commercials and laugh at the slightest things. This is normal and should be embraced as a short deviation from your natural character.

In short, prenatal care is really just living a healthy and balanced life. If you should feel so inclined to also include disease management and screening, that is your right to choose. With that said, we will, in future chapters, address fear. Let's just not call something what it's not. You are the only one responsible for your *Health Care*. A doctor is responsible for catching deviations from normal, not to manage your health. A midwife is there to do both, actually. They are coaches, guides for good health care and observers of potential deviations from normal.

# My Journey Through Birth by Laura:

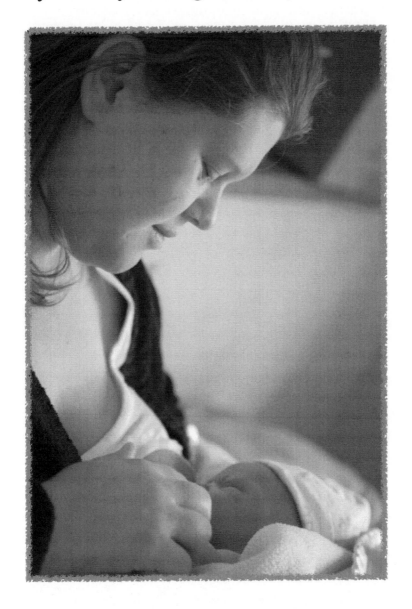

In all honesty, it's difficult to say concisely why I chose to have an unassisted childbirth (UC) at home. My initial journey to UC was complex. Some of the reasons for my choice were religious and spiritual beliefs. Some were emotional issues. Part of my decision had to do with difficulty finding a compatible birth attendant. And yes, part of it was monetary issues. Regardless of my reasons for choosing to have a UC, I'm thankful and feel very blessed for the experience. I will treasure it always.

I'm a pretty private person. Birthing unassisted meant that I was able to do it on my own, without thought as to others' expectations, needs, or fears. There was no risk of iatrogenic injury. I was able to be free from external distractions and allow my instinct and intuition to guide me.

My UCs have had a variety of affects on me. They were both very, very challenging to my integrity. And I don't mean, "Do I tell people my plans, or do I lie?" I mean, I was forced to be fully honest with myself. To face my fears and worries full force. To examine my values and decide, is this something that's *REALLY* important to *ME*? And *WHY*?

These days, I can understand completely why some women just can't or won't consider UC. I had a hospital birth with my first, and then two UCs. (No. No assisted home-births). The first, I had to transfer immediately postpartum. I had thought I'd faced my fears and was prepared to accept all eventualities. I was really shocked and blown away when things didn't go as expected and hoped for. I thought for over a year that I would never be able to face another pregnancy for fear of giving birth (and potentially having something terrible happen). It's challenging to take that responsibility on yourself, knowing that if things go well, it'll be "luck" and if things go poorly, it'll be "all your fault."

Then I got pregnant with my third. I very, very seriously considered having a planned cesarean. Ultimately I decided for another unassisted pregnancy and birth, but with the expectation that I might decide I *NEEDED* to transfer. I knew I needed to be okay with the outcome, *NO MATTER WHAT HAPPENED*. Thankfully nothing went wrong. But the postpartum phase was pretty hard on me. (The whole pregnancy was *VERY* challenging for me, emotionally and physically.) Even though my labor was quick, I was completely drained, in a way that I hadn't been with my girls. I couldn't take care of myself, and my husband couldn't seem to meet my needs. I couldn't go 3 yards to the bathroom on my own the first day. Then I got sick at 3 days postpartum. It took me a long, long time to recover. I got through it, obviously, but if I could do it again, I would have *INSISTED* that my husband call

61

a local midwife or doula to help me within a few hours of the birth. I was in really bad shape. I never expected the need to be waited on hand and foot after having a baby.

My fourth baby was born April 08, also unassisted. Once again, it was a challenging emotional journey. I was forced to dig deep and find the tools to cope with pain, fear, and uncertainty. My husband and I worked hard to communicate about wants, needs, and anxieties so that we could work together as partners. Towards the end of the pregnancy, we thought that I would need an emergency cesarean, which meant I had to work through many issues surrounding surgical birth, empowered choices, and responsibility.

I imagine the value of unassisted birth varies from one individual to the next, but for me, it was a spiritual and emotional journey, making me a stronger and more empowered mother.

*Nova is born:*

March 27, 2002 was one of the most amazing days of my life. My second baby girl, Nova Gabriella Austin, was born at 10:08 AM into her daddy's arms. I think giving birth to Nova was one of the hardest things I've ever done. However, now that some of the post-birth amnesia has kicked in, it also feels like one of the most rewarding things I've ever done. (Though I do remember enough to know that I never want to do *THAT* again!)

I woke up on the 27th very early, around 2:30 AM or so. I went to the bathroom and realized I was having contractions. It was immediately clear that I was not going back to bed just yet. I set up a space in the living room to labor in, thinking everything would probably peter out by the time the sun was up. It was quite lovely. I sat or leaned on my birth ball, rocking and moaning, or just breathing. My candles were lit and I had classical music playing. I checked my cervix and it didn't seem to be dilated at all. This was sort of discouraging as I'd thought I was 1-2 around 32 weeks when my prodromal labor started. Nick arrived home from work at 3:30 AM. He'd had some sort of crisis that I'd encouraged him to stay and get resolved. He asked if I was in labor. "Go to bed," I said. I didn't want to talk, I wanted to go down inside myself, alone.

Time passed. I started feeling hungry around 4:30 AM. I had a banana and stuck some homemade mini-pizzas in the oven. Finally, the pizzas were cooked and I started to munch on them. I got maybe halfway through one and had to rush to the bathroom. Okay, no problem. I empty my bowels. Pretty soon I start to feel nauseous. Am I gonna throw up? I'm not sure, but grab a (relatively) clean waste basket. I don't want to have to put my head in the toilet! Not five minutes later I sat down on the toilet and threw up. Okay. So yeah, this could be it.

Fifteen minutes or so elapsed and I noticed some bloody show. Yay! This is awesome! I'm doing so great; this is easy. I'm smiling and feeling good. I feel encouraged that something is actually happening. My confidence in myself is growing, and I'm really enjoying my labor.

It's probably 6 AM now, and I'm starting to feel hot and sweaty. Pretty gross, actually. So, into the shower I go. I press against the wall and moan, visualizing my cervix opening. At one point, I feel a small gush of fluid and think, "Was that my waters? Nah... Couldn't be, there wasn't enough fluid. Must have just peed." I note that whatever it was seemed to be clear, cause I couldn't see any color. I'm pretty sure that it was my membranes breaking though, because that's the point at which everything starting getting pretty surreal.

Unfortunately, the shower did *NOT* last long enough for me. I noticed the water was not as hot as I wanted it, so I climbed out and went to wake Nick up. I needed him to go find the hot water heater and turn the temp *ALL* the way up! The poor tired guy gets up, goes downstairs and then comes back up and climbs back into bed. I'm thinking, "Umm... Hello?! I'm in labor here!" However, I'm feeling pretty out of it, so I don't say anything.

I never do get back into the shower. I stay in the bathroom, sometimes sitting on the toilet, sometimes squatting, sometimes standing. I'm feeling pretty uncomfortable and vocalizing *LOUDLY*. I start feeling scared and briefly contemplate going to the hospital. I'm at the point of no return, so it's time to look inside myself, say a little prayer, and make a decision. I decide that I'm OK, I'm just overwhelmed by the *INTENSITY* of it all. There's nothing that *MAN* can do for me, except drug me up and/or cut on me. I am the one who has to deliver this baby, nobody else can do it for me.

Around 7:30 AM I start feeling pushy and panicked. I'm in the bathroom and just start *SCREAMING* to Nick (aka Forrest), "*FORREST!!! I NEED YOU RIGHT NOW!!!*" In no time at all, he's there by me, telling me I'm doing great, that everything is wonderful. He was amazing, everything I could have hoped he'd be. I did some pushing here and there, primarily at the peak of the contractions. I couldn't stop myself, so I focused on the belief that my body wouldn't let me hurt myself if I listened to it. Ultimately, my ability to stay home and birth my baby myself was based on my belief that the Creator perfectly capable of birthing, and s/he would get me through it.

Most of the next few hours are a blur to me now. I'm pretty sure I was in transition at this point, and it felt as if it were taking

*FOREVER.* I remember crying that I was scared, I couldn't do it, I just wanted "it" out of me. I wanted it to stop, I wanted the pain to go away. I was afraid, there seemed like a lot of blood. I was very loud, because it felt so intense, I truly didn't know if I could handle it. I seriously contemplated going to the hospital to ask for a c-section. (I did dismiss the thought pretty quickly though, but it sounded pretty good at the time.) Birthing is hard work! No wonder they call it "labor!"

Finally, I got the break I'd been sobbing for. I was sitting on the toilet with a warm compress and found the courage to reach inside and feel for the baby's head. I wanted to know how close "he" was. Elation! Right there, just past my second knuckle. It was the most incredible thing I've ever felt. Excitedly I exclaimed, "I can feel the baby's head!" Nick moaned in response, "Oh Wow!" I could also feel the edge of the amniotic sac, though I didn't realize what it was at the time.

I'm starting to push more in earnest, and it feels like it's going *SO* **SLOWLY**! I say as much to Nick... "It's taking too long, she's not coming!" Of course, she was coming, it just felt like forever. My expectations didn't include what felt like such long, drawn out intensity. Today, it makes me smile to remember how convinced I was that my labor was never going to end.

Finally, as I stood with one leg up on the toilet, the baby began to crown. Oh man, it burns! *WOW*! I feel like I'm being stretched to my limits. I tell Nick I'm going to tear in front, I need the hot compress there, he disagrees. He thinks that if I'm going to tear, it'll be "in back." (Later he told me that my perineum was all white and he was sure I was going to tear.)

At this point, time has no meaning to me. I bear down hard and finally get the head out. What a relief! Nick used a clean rag and wiped out Nova's mouth. He tells me I can push again. I think, "*SHIT!* I am pushing!" It feels like an eternity has passed. (In reality, it was only about a minute.) I ask if either of the shoulders are out. (I'm not actually having a contraction, I'm just trying to push like hell because I want to get Nova out of inside me and into my arms!) "No," comes the reply. A feeling of dread settles on me. My biggest fear was the possibility of shoulder dystocia, an extremely rare but incredibly dangerous circumstance where the shoulders get stuck behind the pubic bone.

A contraction finally builds up and I exclaim, "She's coming!" And she does come... Both shoulders at once! Wow! Everything that followed her delivery is a blur to me now... I remember stepping over her cord and Nick handing her to me. Him saying he's going to pass out, and laying down on the floor outside the bathroom. Me exclaiming, "She's breathing!" and "It's a girl!" and wanting to cry at the sheer joy and intensity of it all. I remember saying,

"Welcome Baby Nova" and "Come on now" and "I love you." I kissed her and rubbed her chest and legs because her breathing was somewhat grunty and her color was poor.

I wish that I could end the story by saying, "Thankfully, she pinked right up. I birth the placenta, we cut her cord, washed up, and climbed into bed to nurse." Unfortunately, that's not how it went. Before she was born, Nick noticed meconium in the waters, and called 911 with my unhappy consent. Apparently the call didn't go through the way it should have, because after she was born, they still had not arrived. He called them again.

I sat on the toilet and realized the placenta was coming. Nick got me a glass bowl to birth it into. I was relieved to have delivered it before the EMTs arrived. I'd felt nervous they might put traction on the cord, causing me to bleed. Still, I felt concerned that Nova was so sleepy. Wasn't she supposed to want to nurse right off? I guess she was all tuckered out from being born!

EMTs arrived 20-30 minutes after the birth while I was sitting in the bathtub. They checked her over, cut her cord. We were both taken to UCSF to get check out. Nova's lungs were clear, thankfully, which meant she hadn't aspirated any meconium. Yay Daddy for getting it all out! Meconium isn't automatically an emergency complication, but it can sometimes mean that baby is in distress. Since Nick wasn't prepared to deal with possible MAS (meconium aspiration syndrome), it's understandable that he wanted someone else there who definitely would know what to do.

To make a long story shorter, we spent about 30 hours in the hospital. For the most part, it went pretty well. It wasn't how I had wanted the first two days of my baby's life to go, that's how life goes sometimes. I'm home with my perfect baby girl, and she's safe and healthy.

When I think of Nova's birth, I am filled with such intense emotions. While it felt so gloriously right, I also recognize how dreadfully terrible it could have turned out. There are so many things that might have happened. Death happens, birth happens, it's all a part of life. Babies die in the hospital, babies die at home. Most people don't ever really face that reality. We don't want to face it as a reality.

By birthing at home, I was able to listen to my body, to give myself over to the birth. I experienced the intensity of pure, raw birth. I truly felt between the worlds. It exhilarated me; it terrified me. I felt as if it was too much for a mere mortal to experience. I feel aged, like I've seen the Deity and lived to tell the tale. And I thank God for that experience. I've been blessed.

*Elliot is born:*

It's been more than three weeks now since my son was born. I try to put the experience into words so that I may share it with others, but find that I cannot. Like my second daughter, Nova, my son was born unassisted, at home. I made the decision to birth without medical attendants both times after a great deal of prayer, meditation, and no small amount of uncertainty.

The first time I decided to give birth unassisted, I *KNEW* it was the right choice, though it was a difficult decision because I was the only one in my life who really knew that. Intuitively, I felt sure that if I gave birth in a hospital, something very, very bad would happen. I don't believe this was just fear. I didn't have that feeling with my first daughter (hospital born) or my son. During that birth, we had some "complications" that, thankfully, resolved without major incident. However, I feel certain that things would have turned from bad to worse very rapidly had we been in a hospital.

When I became pregnant with my son, I didn't have those strong feelings about giving birth at home versus in the hospital. Instead, I had a tremendous amount of *FEAR*. Fear of birth, fear of pain, fear of persecution, and above all, fear of death. I was afraid of a big baby, of my baby getting stuck and dying, of transporting to the hospital where who-knows what kind of drama would ensue. I was afraid something would go terribly wrong and I would lose my children, my husband, my self- everything. I seriously considered a planned cesarean section. It was the only way, I felt, to be sure that my baby didn't get stuck being born.

Ultimately, I decided that my fears were just that: fears. I opted to have my baby at home, prepared to the very best of my ability. I mentally prepared myself to the possibility of transferring, facing and accepting that fear, and then I moved on to preparing for the birth I hoped to have. I visualized the different ways I might labor and birth, the ways I would cope with fears and sensations, how I might breath. I said affirmations and practiced relaxation techniques when my anxiety threatened to overwhelm me. I printed out affirmations and taped them to my computer monitor and desk, and bought a laminated affirmation poster and taped in my bathroom. I prayed. And somehow, I knew. Everything would be okay. My fears were still there, but deep inside, I knew that it would all work out the way it was meant to. I trusted.

Those nine months felt like an eternity as they were passing. It seemed as if I would never give birth, and part of me hoped it was so. The other part of me, of course, was ready to be *DONE*. The fatigue, the sore hips and pelvis, the insomnia, the inability to roll over! Finally, December began. I had deliberately avoided handing out one "definitive" due date, although I knew the date that I would most likely be hitting was the 40 week mark. I felt certain that I *WOULD NOT* give birth on that date; I would give birth earlier (I hoped), or later (I believed).

I grew antsy as the days passed. I had bouts of contractions, pre-labor, diarrhea, nesting. Each time I would think, 'soon'. Soon. But another day would pass. December 9th, I made plans to go out shopping with a friend two evenings later. I went home that evening, put my two year old to bed, and treated myself to a movie, popcorn, and red raspberry leaf tea. My husband brought home some peanut M&Ms at my request. During all this, I had sporadic, very infrequent contractions. Yet they were different. I had odd twinges inside my vagina. Not cervical, something odd, different. My thought changed from "Soon," to "Maybe..." And as I prepared to go to bed for the night, I was seized with horror that my baby might possibly be born in the disaster that was our bedroom. It had to be clean, de-cluttered, packed! (We were supposed to be moving in a week and a half.)

A few hours later, very little had been accomplished, and I was still not having regular contractions. Just odd twinges inside me that begged to be pushed upon. So I made love to my dear husband in a strange place of surrender and trust. He fell asleep around 2:00 AM, knowing that I was having contractions, but not knowing where I was with them. I wanted him to sleep. I wanted to be alone for a while, and I felt sure that it would be many hours before my baby was born, if my contractions didn't peter out on me again. I wandered around the house for a little while, laboring, before getting into a candle lit bath.

From here, it seems there is very little to say. At 3:05 AM, my water exploded with a loud pop and a gush. It was shocking, I think to both me and my little guy, who squirmed all over the place inside of me. I had still been in denial, a bit, but I knew now, it was on. There was no turning back.

I got out to set up the last of my birthing supplies and post a quick note online that my water had broken and I was in labor. More water gushed out with the next contraction, soaking the towel I was sitting on and the carpet beneath my exercise ball. It didn't take long before I got back into the bathtub.

My vocalizations began getting loud around 4 AM, and woke up my husband. He quietly came in to see how things were going. I was getting pushy, but couldn't seem to explain that, or even really comprehend the fact myself. I was beyond intellectual thought. I told him I wanted to go to the hospital and get drugs. He suggested we wait 15 minutes. This somehow made sense to me, so I waited. And I soon began to push in earnest. And push, and push. And ever so slowly, in my dark, warm bathroom, my son's wrinkly head began to emerge. It was as normal as taking a shit, but my Lord! I've never taken a shit that big. I also experienced the "ring of fire" that is described in so many birth books and stories, but had experienced only briefly myself in my previous births.

Then, his head was born! Finally! He began to move and squirm inside of me, and his arm was born, and then his other arm and shoulders and, finally, he "swam" out into our bathtub, into the world. It was 5:05 AM, exactly two hours after my water had broken and I had accepted that my baby was going to be born. December 10th, 2004, my due date! Elliott Maxwell, my son.

Within an hour, I was in bed, nursing both my brand new baby and my two year old. Soon my six year old woke up and came to meet her new brother. It was so simple and basic, yet I feel like there are a million tiny details too intimate and sacred to share. It was the way it was meant to be.

I have three amazing children now; two daughters and a son. Twice I have lost little ones very early in pregnancy. Each of these souls have taught me so much. I am beyond grateful to have had them as a part of my journey. Each pregnancy, each birth, each milestone we reach together changes me, changes who I am as a woman and a mother. Each time I give birth, it seems that I am reborn. With each rebirth comes change. I am changed, my children, my husband, my extended family are all changed. My relationship with myself and the Divine is changed. I am blessed and thankful.

In my selfishness, I want to keep my story and experience to and for myself, to savor it. Still, I will share what I can articulate in the hope that my experiences will help to inspire positive growth, change, and thought in my extended circle of friends and acquaintances. May it leave you as blessed as it has me.

Addendum: He was a big baby, but birth worked! He did not get stuck on his way out. He weighed in at 10 lbs 9 ozs on his third day of life, the day my milk came it. He most likely was at least 11 lbs at birth, possibly as much as 12 pounds! (Most babies lose roughly 10% of their body weight the first two-three days.) He was 21 inches long and his head circumference was 14 inches.

*Mira Evangeline is born:*

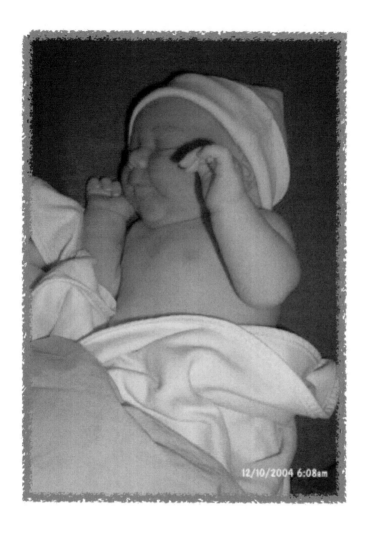

12/10/2004 6:08am

Yesterday morning, at 6:14 AM, she was born into her mommy and daddy's hands at *HOME!* I had resolved to go to the hospital after all the drama and fear at the ultrasound clinic. However, when I went into labor, none of the "clues" that true labor had begun until it was *FAR* too late to leave. I don't think I would have even gotten to the van in time.

The short version of the birth story: On the evening of the 9th, I warned my husband to go to bed early. I wasn't having regular contractions or anything, but if my past pattern held, I would go into labor in the wee hours of the morning if he stayed up late. True to my pattern, when he came to bed after midnight, I woke up and was hit with an intense contraction. A few minutes later, another, and I decided to get up and enjoy my "birth pool" since I wouldn't get to give birth in it (I had resolved to head to the hospital once labor was well established).

In the pool, I shifted position, and gradually, began to doze between contractions. Since I've typically had at least one bout of hard "practice labor," I was certain things would peter out, and this belief was reinforced by the fact that I was falling asleep! Plus there was no rhyme or reason to the pattern of contractions, no bloody show, and no broken waters.

At 5:45 AM, I went to the bathroom. I had a strong contraction and at the peak, felt pushy! "Uhhh..." It was *WAY* too soon for that. I did *NOT* want to risk swelling my cervix when I could not possibly be even remotely close to giving birth. I would get in the pool again and the contractions would stop. Shit, the pool had cooled off way too much, and needed to be partially drained. As soon as the next contraction, I practically ran up the stairs to sit on the toilet in the master bathroom. I whimpered to my dear husband, "Nick..." I panted a little. "I need your help." He woke up and did as I asked- start draining the pool so it could be refilled. So, you know, my contractions would stop, lol! 'Cause I was done with this stupid bout of "false labor."

I went down the stairs again and went on my hands and knees for a contraction where I began to freak out, begging my husband to "*MAKE IT STOP!*" We all know what that means, of course? Yep, serious transition time. It was at this point I had to realize, this baby was on the way, and I wasn't going anywhere. I sat on the toilet and the baby started coming down. As in, *OUT!* I could not move, and had a moment of panic that she would fall into the toilet. No worries. I guided her head halfway out, and cried about how much it hurt. Then there was a short pause and I was able to come forward into a hands and knees/ crouch so my husband could help catch. And out she came! Just that fast.

Even though Drs had suspected Intra Uterine Growth Retardation, she was well! Mira Evangeline, tiny and perfect with great strong lungs and petite little fingers and toes and a round fuzzy head. Contrary to the ominous predictions, she was a good sized newborn at *7 lbs 14 ozs!* Perfectly proportioned, and no signs of being in distress at all.

Our Journey through birth by Nicole:

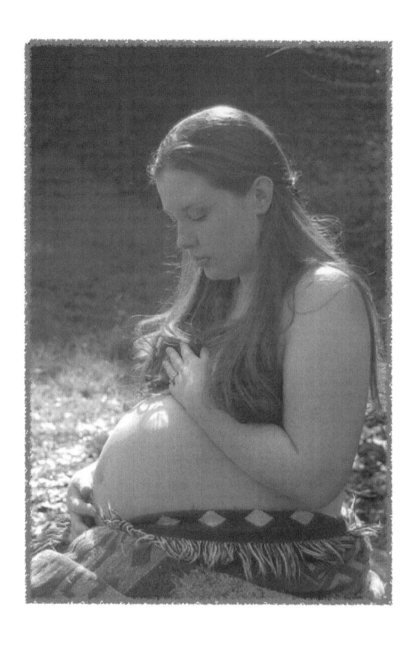

After my daughter's hospital birth, I knew that I wanted something

different for my second child. Something that felt real. Something that I could hold with me for the rest of my life. To always be able to look back and say, "I did that," and be proud. My path towards an unassisted pregnancy and birth felt natural and fluid. I felt a strong desire to have complete control, since I had given all my power away with Ciara's birth. I desperately wanted and needed it back.

I do not think I have ever prepared myself more for anything in my life than I did for this birth. I wanted to know everything. I completely sunk into birth, and thought for nine months about what I wanted. I read for hours upon hours, and wrote my thoughts down, trying to reach a point where I felt completely ready.

Everyone asked me, "Oh, you must be totally done, right?" I would respond, "No, I'm not ready for this to be over. I want to enjoy these last days," and that was the complete truth. This was my last pregnancy, last baby, last ever. The thought of it just ending so quickly really scared me.

Still, as I drove home from work in the very early hours of Tuesday, April 3, 2007, I felt a twinge in my back. And then another. A quiet excitement began to build inside of me. I knew this was the beginning.

I went home that night, and got ready for bed at about 2 AM. Before I slipped into bed with my husband and daughter, I looked out the window. A full moon shone back at me. I opened the window and stood breathing in the night air with my eyes closed. It was crisp and quite cold, but exhilarating. I realized I was ready for whatever was happening. I left the curtains open for the moonlight to shine in, and I settled into a deep sleep.

I awoke in an uncomfortable state at 7 AM. It took me a few moments to realize that my back was still throbbing. I tried to close my eyes to rest, but the bed quickly became unbearable. I made a trip to the restroom, and was met with bloody show and mucous. This is really it.

I walked about the house cleaning excitedly. I was not really sure what to do next. I knew I should go back to bed, but I wanted my husband to know, since he would be gone until about 5 PM that day at work. I called his work so they could let him know what was going on, in case I needed to get in touch with him again if labor picked up faster than I expected. I then forced myself back to bed, to get all the sleep I could.

My daughter awoke at 10 AM, and was quick to wake me as well. We got in the shower, and I realized I had some errands to run. We got ourselves all ready, both of us in overalls. I put my hair in braided pigtails and was very pleased with myself. "This is really happening!" I kept thinking. We both hopped in the car, and ran up to the library. I had so many books on hold and knew that I would not have another time to pick them up. I talked to a friend before we went inside, and she asked me how far apart my contractions were. I was not having any noticeable stop and start contractions. I just felt really achy, like I was about to start my period, I told her. Then, just as I said that, I felt my uterus tighten. "Wait, there's one..."

We made our way inside, and Ciara ran around playing and coloring in the kid's section. I settled into the rocking chair with a book I just checked out (A Midwife's Story), and tried to read. I kept looking around at all the kids playing and the moms chasing after them and thinking, "They have no idea I'm in labor." It was my fun little secret. I smiled and read a few chapters from my book.

After a quick grocery store trip, where I bought myself tons of yummy food like cakes and soup, we made it home. I made many bathroom visits once we got home, and was greeted by even more mucous and bloody show. I sat and wished my husband was home, so that I could focus a little more on what was going on inside me, instead of my daughter running around squealing and temper tantrum-ing. She was really wild that day, maybe sensing something was going on. Surprisingly, my husband showed up two hours early, with even more cake (I love cake, and he knows it) and a movie. We ran about cleaning, and preparing. I had been putting off doing my belly cast and suddenly realized we needed to get it done or there would not be another chance!

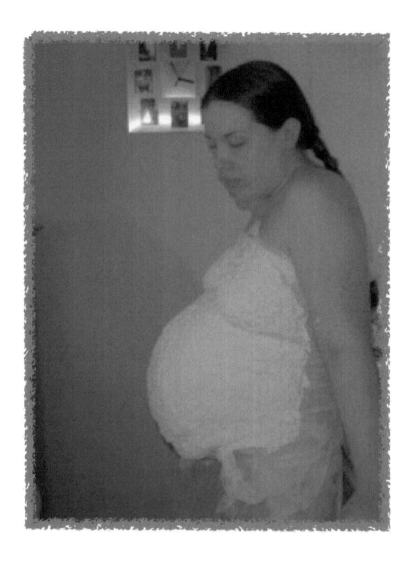

I sat as still as I could, as my husband coated my torso in craft plaster. After almost an hour of not being able to move during contractions, I waddled my way in to get him off the phone and get the "damn cast off of me". I was so incredibly uncomfortable, and once that thing was off, I jumped into the shower to get some relief. Contractions picked up more and were now about 4 minutes apart. I was not clock-watching in the slightest, just merely guesstimating the time in between them. I barely looked at the clock most of the day, actually. I wanted to focus entirely on what my body was telling me.

After my shower, I lay down again to rest and read. Seven o' clock snuck up, and I awoke with stronger contractions. This was about the time that I began to have to really pause and concentrate on the contractions. I wandered out into the house in a bit of a haze. I felt electric and tingly, like I had too much caffeine.

I tested out my birthing ball; it was definitely more comfortable to sit on than anything else around. I bounced around on that for a few hours in between snacking and bathroom breaks. I had even more mucous and bloody show every time I went. I never actually lost a mucous 'plug', I just slimed all day long. I never thought I could create so much mucous. It was a bit uncomfortable and gross, really. But I made sure to report it laughingly to my husband each time I checked.

My sister arrived around 8 PM, as she was there to watch over my daughter whenever labor got too intense. I was then able to make some much needed phone calls. I called my parents to let them know the baby would be coming soon. They frantically said they would be coming over soon. "No! No, that's okay! We're all going to bed soon. You don't want to come over now!" They had wanted to be here during the birth, but all I wanted was a private birth with just my husband and myself. They were appeased when I agreed to call them thirty minutes before I thought the baby would be born. I had no intentions to, and knew they would be too happy to be upset when I called them when it was all done.

I made another phone call to my friend, Veronica, and we chatted for an hour. It was getting late, nearing eleven. She commented about how calm I was acting over the phone, and said it would probably be later the next day. Contractions were about 3 minutes apart now, and I was still feeling good. I got up and made my sister and    husband dinner, and bounced around on my ball for a bit longer. I was noticing that I was having a harder time handling contractions about then. Once one would come on, I would kick my legs around, walk about quickly, and flail my arms. Generally, just toss myself about looking silly.

My sister thought that was pretty amusing, and she chatted with me in the kitchen as I did this birth "dance". I thought how so many women seem calm and natural in labor, reverting to a primal state and knowing what to do. I had thought that I would instinctively know how to handle these in my own way, and I guess I did. I just thought it might be a bit more graceful and little less ridiculous. Still, my jumping about helped. I ate dinner and decided I wanted a change of pace. Maybe a warm bath would bring about this birth goddess?

I ran my bath with some lavender oil, lit some candles, turned the lights out and got in. As my body entered the bath, the water rose almost to the brim. I lay down on my side, with half of my body under the water, and listened to the water drain out slowly. I spent a good hour or more, laying on one side, then the other, and listening to the water flow out. When it cooled, I would turn the tap with my foot, filling it up to the top again. My mind was filled with the sound of the water draining, and I imagined it to be a river.

Brian peeped in every so often, asking if I needed anything. I wanted my birth CD my friend Trish made, but he could not find his CD player. He ran about trying to set up this larger stereo in the bathroom. In between his frantic footsteps, my contractions took a turn. I felt the baby move down, into my pelvis. I felt a widening. A sharpness. Again and again. Once Brian had set the stereo completely up, I asked him to get me out .... now.

The contractions were quickening and I could not get out on my own anymore. Getting me out of the tub was an event, as we had to time them in between contractions, and I was so big, and the tub so, so small. When I finally made it out, the water dipped to just a few inches high. "Geez, I must be huge," I thought.

The bathroom was moist and dark. I stood there, not knowing what to do next. I did not want to leave the warmth, but the room felt too hard to labor in. I stood still, as the contractions rolled in and out. My husband just stood beside me in the dark, unsure of what I wanted. "I don't know what to do, Brian." I spoke to him in between the ever-intensifying pains, hanging onto the towel rack.

I thought I would know what to do. Where was this primal birth power that I was supposed to be reverting to? I felt confused, and my mind blanked between each contraction. I only had time to recover before another would come. I kept waiting for some strong sense to come to me, some voice to tell me where to go to have my baby. I listened quietly and heard nothing. Another contraction. Then another. I gripped Brian, naked and dripping wet.

He led me to the bedroom. I stood for a while, just trying to handle the contractions as they came faster and faster. I held onto him so tightly, and he to me. I began to weep quietly, though without tears, during each contraction. They were so incredibly intense, the power of it all just made me weak. All I could think of was how I wanted to lay down and sleep. But then I would remind myself that it would soon be over. That I was strong, and could make it. I just needed to hang on. It would not be much longer, I knew.

I never checked my dilation, as I wanted to fully listen to my body and not become dismayed if labor progressed different from what I expected. I felt wetness dripping down my legs. I took a towel, and wiped. Blood showed bright red. I knew I could not labor much longer on my feet, so I had Brian get me some pillows and I got on my hands and knees, with the pillows under my chest.

Contractions came faster and faster. I felt every inch of the pain, down into my legs, up my back, into my bones. I thought, "Where is this natural pain relief everyone speaks of? Why am I not in a daze?!" I hugged the pillows beneath me and Brian rubbed my back calmly. I cried out from the pain, wishing for it to be over soon.

Suddenly, waves of nausea swept over me. "Good! Transition. It's almost over!" I thought. Brian got me a bowl, but I never threw up. I was overwhelmed with the contractions, when suddenly I felt pushy. I tried to hold it back, but my body forced me to bear down. I did what I was being led to do, and suddenly my water burst all over the bed. I felt pressure and pain moving farther down. So much pain.

My body was forcing me to push more now, but I was not ready. I tried to hold myself back. I had thought when women spoke of their body pushing on its own, that it was from the inside. Instead, I was actively pushing, bearing down, as my mind screamed, "Stop it! Not so fast! Let it just happen!" It was as if my mind was completely cut off from my body. My thoughts ran quickly, as I attempted to deal with this new issue. I repeated aloud, "Calm down calm down calm down..." Over and over.

I was slowly able to regain control a few times. I breathed in and out loudly, holding my body back, and suddenly I would be pushing and pushing and pushing! I could barely breathe between the extreme bearing down I was doing. I felt the baby move farther and farther down. The pressure became so intense. I have no idea where Brian was at this point. I could only attempt to hold myself back. Such an inner battle I have never experienced! Body versus mind.

I was now lying on my stomach, somehow. I had lost the strength to retain the hands and knees position. I was sweaty. Soaking wet, actually. I could barely lift myself. Brian said to me, "I can see something. I don't know what it is, but it looks good!" At that point, I just relinquished all my power to my body, and was swept away in the pushing. There was burning. Oh, the burning! Brian oiled me up, but I honestly could not feel anything besides the intensity of the baby pushing through. Wider and wider, until I thought I would break open.

"There's the head! Hold on..." Brian said as he unwrapped the cord. "There you go..."

A beautiful wetness fell from me.

Silence for a moment.

"Come on, baby!"

Gurgles, splutters and cries erupted. Our baby cried out for the first time. I felt such an intense relief, more than anything I imagine relief could feel like. It was done. I had done it. The baby was here!

I turned around and caught my first glimpse.

He was here.

"You have a son!" Brian exclaimed.

I turned myself, maneuvered the cord and then he was in my arms. So fresh, new. I smelled him, and took him in deeply. This was the reality I had been seeking for so long. This is what I gave up when I had my daughter. Life erupting in front of me.

Ciara cried out from the other end of the house. She had been asleep, but the cries awoke her. She came in, looking sleepy-eyed, but soon jumped up and down, squealing, "Baby! What's that baby?!" My sister, Sara, called out that he was born at 3:23 AM. She had woken up the last few minutes of labor and listened from the living room.

We all sat together on the bed as a family, admiring him, and talking excitedly. I sat up and passed the placenta after about thirty minutes. Ciara screamed out, "What is *THAT*?! I'm going to see Sara!" She came back in and repeated over and over, "I don't like that. That's gross. Blah!" Brian and I laughed at her disapproval of the placenta. I examined it, looking it over closely. It was warm, bloody, and heavy. My hands were coated in blood. In fact, I was covered all over. I left to take a quick shower, and once back, we decided on his first name. A name had not been chosen, since we both wanted to wait and see how we felt after the baby was born. Oliver was the first name that came to both of us.

And so ends this part of my life. It came and went so fast, I barely had time to register what had happened. I could not have asked for a better, more perfect birth. It was exactly as I had envisioned, the day and the night. The darkness. Just Brian and me, and our baby coming so quickly in the night.

I will now be able to take those moments with me for the rest of my life, and now I can say that I did that. I took full responsibility for my body and baby. I listened to what my body was naturally meant to do, and trusted in it. I gave myself up to the strength that was inside of me. Such an experience should never be withheld from any woman. This is what life is. There's nothing else that compares.

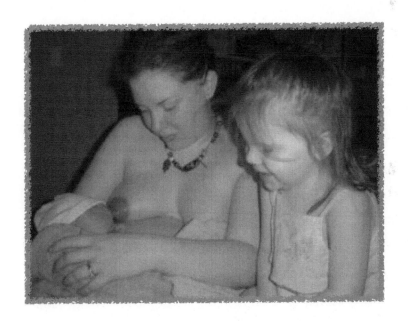

# Our Journey Through Birth by Marisa:

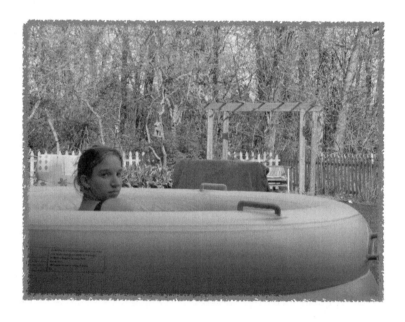

It was on Beltane, May day, your due date. I was never a believer of "due dates" and whenever people asked when you were due, I told them springtime.

You came earth-side on such a beautiful, warm day. The trees were just starting to blossom with little buds. I could feel the twinge of labor coming on, slowly and lightly. I told my dear partner, Jesse, that it was time, and we drove to a friend's farm.

When we arrived, I was just in the mood to take a slow amble around the farm. We walked on a tiny dirt path through the tall grass to a little pond surrounded by huge trees and flowers. The contractions slowed down. I guess the rocking sensation of walking relaxed you. We slept outside on the grass under a tree for most of the afternoon.

I woke up with the urge to go take a warm bath. Jesse and I got into the bathtub and I felt so relaxed...and then the contractions started rushing in with gusto. Blood was coming out in little bits. Jesse told the midwives that things were really progressing. They got on their way, and we filled up the big blue birthing tub outside on the grass. I absolutely loved the smell of fresh grass and watched two little spring robins twitter around.

The rushes became stronger and stronger. Soon, I lost nearly all my sense of control and just let go. I let the sounds inside of me out. I moved around with every pang of contraction. Our midwives came outside to check on your heartbeat once in every while. They were completely silent and stayed inside most of the time. It was starting to get dark and cold outside. I asked my midwife when she came outside, "When will I know how or when to push?" She smiled and said that my body would do it for me, and that you and I would work together.

Not very long after that, I decided to head into the bathroom with Jesse. I took a few sips of water, and with three *absolutely* overwhelming contractions, I yelled and felt like I was about to throw up. I felt like I was being turned inside out. There was absolutely no holding back. You came so FAST. I was standing up. Jesse could see the intact water bag come out first, your head twisting out. The bag broke and you slid right out, in your father's hands.

Jesse immediately gave you to me. You raised your arm towards me, your fingers spread out, touching my heart.

And then I realized that your birth was unhindered and beautiful. The way women in so many cultures have done it for centuries. I felt empowered........And the rain immediately started pouring outside.

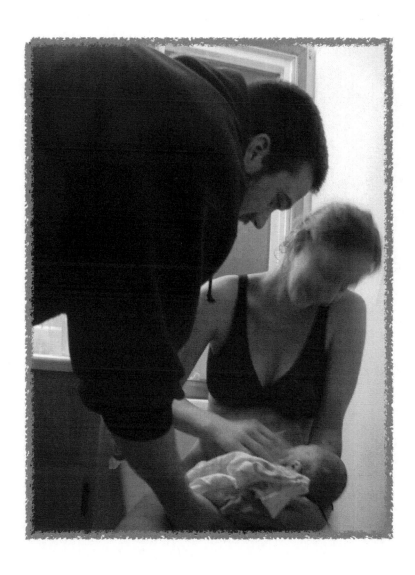

# Psychological Care

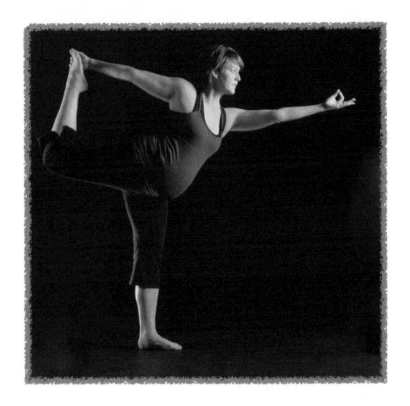

Through my training as a child birth educator and through my training as a yoga teacher, but mostly through my experiences in life school, I have learned one of the greatest lessons: That is that if our mental state is not nurtured and cared for, it will impact every area of our lives in a negative way. Pregnancy is a heightened time of growth and expansion and not just in a physical sense. A woman will find that during pregnancy and birth, she is tested in her views of herself as a woman and even simply a human in this world. With her increased emotional sensitivity, it seems that there are often issues that she is facing and needing to think and feel her way through. When a woman has reached the understanding that she is simply more emotionally sensitive at this stage in her life, it can make these processes easier, but it does not eliminate the need to respond to the 'issues' that take center stage for her.

Pregnancy can be a time where a woman suddenly feels consumed by very important life decisions, like 'will I work or will I stay home?', and 'will I breast feed and how do I feel about that?'. Those are just a couple of the big ones and it seems that at every turn, a pregnant woman is making big decisions at a time when making decisions becomes more difficult. I've found some of the exercises that I have learned have been very helpful and here I share some tips and tricks to help you be healthy and balanced in your mental state.

•If you feel like crying, do it. The whole point of tears is to rid your body of stress hormones. If you do not shed the tears that want to come, then you will become overloaded with stress hormones which might make the next issue that rises even larger an issue than it really is simply because you are hormonally constipated!

•If you feel like laughing, do it. Laughing is one of the healthiest things you can do. There are even laughing groups out there.

While I'm not suggesting that you join one necessarily, I am suggesting that this time of heightened sensitivity to emotion should be taken advantage of. The laughing is good for both you and your baby, so lighten up! Don't be so serious.

•Journal. This is a time more full of thoughts and feelings than any other in your life will likely be. Journaling allows a person to process thought and feel mentally purged. Don't worry about your writing skills. This is just for you.

•If you really feel that you are struggling with some deep and potentially buried thoughts and feelings, write with your non-dominant hand. This will literally open up the locked doors. You may write about things that you thought you were 'over' and this will allow you to release the buried emotions.

•Be creative and artistic. Try drawing, coloring, sewing or clay molding. Taping into your creative side is doubly healthy while pregnant as this is a time for heightened creativity. A woman is more tightly tied to her creative and nurturing qualities at this time in life. If there is an art that you gravitate toward, let yourself indulge and express it.

•Make friends that are pregnant and like-minded. Join groups, attend meetings, and more. Ask your midwife or doctor, if you have one, what groups that you can join. If you are going unassisted, contact a midwife or doula to find out what is going on in your local community. The support of like-minded individuals is powerful and can bring a measure of peace to your choices.

•Talk. This falls in line with the previous. Find a friend or confidant that you can talk with about everything that you are experiencing. For some, this is their partner. Some don't have that relationship. Either way, a person who will listen and give input and feed back is very valuable.

•While these are just touching on the important aspects of psychological care, I would recommend a book called *Creating a Joyful Birth Experience* by Lucia Capacchione and Sandra Bardsley. And, the book *Birthing From Within* by Pam England and Rob Horowitz. The exercises in these books will take you deeper into the tips and tricks listed above. It is just as essential to the health of you and your baby to tend to your psychological care as it is your physical care. Emotions left unexpressed will manifest themselves in your body, your pregnancy, your labor, and your birth.

# My Journey Through Birth by Tralee:

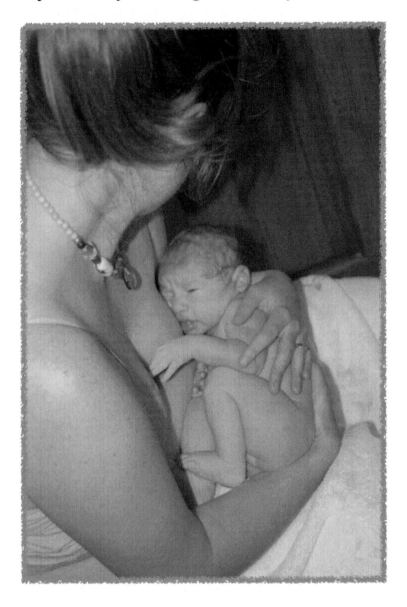

*Valkyrie Vola Knapp is born, 11- 21-07:*

With my first child, I was 6 days past her estimated due date. I was getting very anxious. We had an OBGYN appointment at 1:00 PM on the 20th. I was dilated maybe a centimeter. The OB said she wasn't worried and that she would probably see me in a few days with a baby in my arms. As we were driving to meet my parents I felt an interesting sensation, like a pressure and it got my attention enough just to think 'hum, I wonder what that was.' Little did I know this was what a contraction felt like. I was able to talk and walk around during them; they slowly increased in frequency over the next hour or so. They got closer together and a little stronger. I was excited; this is what I was waiting for. I was able to grab a bite to eat as we headed down to a store about 25 miles south of town. We were there about an hour and things were definitely progressing.

We decided to head home, get comfortable because this was it. It was around 4:30 PM when we arrived at home. So I had been having contractions for a good 4 hours. My husband and I decided we would go to the hospital when they were 2 min apart lasting for 1 min. So I walked around the house. Sitting still or lying down didn't feel as good. So every time I felt a contraction I got up and walked around the room. This continued till my contractions reached the point we talked about (2 min apart) it was a little past 10 PM when we drove to the hospital. I got all checked in, I remember being very calm and quiet during the contractions.

The nurses said I couldn't be that far along because I was being too quiet. I was focused on each contraction.

As I settled into the birthing room the nurses joked "If you could have this baby before our shift is over that would be great. It is a pain trying to do a shift change during active labor." The pattern of the contractions being 2 min apart lasting about 1 min continued for about another 6 hours, made for a long night. The night was a blur. I remember trying to take a bath, throwing up, and lots of pacing around the hospital room. They said they had a hospital rule that that they had to monitor me every ½ hour for 15 min, or something like that. I would only let them use an external fetal monitor. I still hated it. I was strapped to a machine and forced to stare at this monitor showing me each contraction approaching like a wave about to crash over me on a beach, but I wasn't allowed to run away. A few times I had to tell them "no, please don't hook me up to that, I need to walk around." The staff was good about respecting my wishes for a non-invasive, natural birth.

I remember looking at the clock and seeing it read 3 AM and felt like the night would never end. I was getting tired, and later I kneeled down on the chair in the room facing a window that overlooked the city and the creek down below and all of a sudden felt like bearing down. When the nurses came back in I told them what I felt and they checked me, I was only at a 7 cm. They told me I know you want to push but try not to, you are not fully

104

dilated and we don't want you to injure yourself. Telling a woman in labor not to push, yeah right! They called the doctor on call to let them know I was getting close.

All of a sudden I pushed and it felt like I peed, when in fact my water had broken. They had me on the bed lying on my side trying to hold back the pushing. It was so hard; all I wanted to do was push the baby out. Soon they were on the phone to the OB saying they didn't think they could hold me back anymore. And about 30 min later the doctor came rolling in with everything, she sat down on a stool at the foot of the bed, they rolled me over and up and as my legs separated my husband yelled "Oh my God, Tralee, I can see her head." I did feel a little burning sensation during the pushes and I remember the sounds I made. Oh my, they didn't sound human, so deep and low. I gave a few good pushes and Valkyrie was in my arms. I was shocked.

The doctor barely made it, she literally only had time to sit down and then there the baby was! The after birth was fast; I placed my baby girl right on my chest and began to nurse her. I laid there holding her for a good 30 min and then handed her off to my husband. There was a little repairing that needed to be done, I had torn slightly but nothing bad. It was amazing. As I was recovering I turned to the nurses and said "Well we got it done before your shift was over." We all had a good laugh. When the new nurse came in to move us to our room she looked at me and said "I hear you are a Rockstar". "Me, why is that?", I asked. She said she had been working there 20 years and I was the first person to come in with a birth plan and follow it to a T. I felt proud. We were moved to recovery and I drifted off to sleep with my baby girl in my arms. The rest is history. (The total labor was about 17 hours long.)

*Skyler Sierra Knapp is born, July 13, 2009.*

Giving birth to my first born had gone so well. No interventions and 100% natural that when we got pregnant with our second I looked at my husband and said "Can we do this one at home?" He was completely on board. This is her story:

Skyler Sierra Knapp was born on July 13th 2009 at about 4:57 AM. (I really don't know the exact moment I held that beautiful little baby in my arms, but I do remember hearing the chime of my husband's grandmother's clock ring 5 shortly after I was holding her.)

Skyler had a wonderful birth. The contractions began around 1 PM on the 12th. They were short, infrequent and uneventful. So we walked all around downtown Salem. It began to get cool and windy, so we headed back to the car and went for a drive. A thunderstorm moved in and soon it was thunder, lightning and pouring rain. The contractions were still uneventful so we kept on driving. Around 5 PM, we made our way back home. The contractions were getting constant so we got set for a night at home. We even had a few friends over to knit and watch "Flight of the Conchords" We sent them home about 10 PM...who knows how long this labor would be and we thought we'll call them back over when it gets exciting. My first child, Valkyrie went to bed and the rest of the night was a bit of a blur. I called our Midwife and she said to call her back when the contractions were 4 min apart and lasting about 1 min. I remember when we called our Midwife and her apprentice to say the contractions were about 4 min apart for the last 30 min. They rushed over to our house and we there about 11 PM.

The house was quiet and we had nice music playing, candles burning and low lights. It was beautiful! The hours slowly passed with each one progressing just a little bit more, it was turning out a lot like Valkyrie's birth; easy but long. Yes, I said easy. To me birth is natural, not painful...yeah a little discomfort but every contraction was helping me, every moment was me experiencing me. I looked forward to each new phase, like a runner trains for a marathon...after so much prep and training you think, "yeah come on, bring it...bring on that hill, I can do this." Jeff, my husband, was there by my side the whole time, coaching me along the way. I used one of those large yoga balls to lean over and rest all my weight on during the contractions. I was in the position of hands and knees a lot. Our Midwife was checking the baby's heart rate about every hour and she was sounding great. I tried to lay down in bed once and sleep a little but as soon as the contraction came it was a hard one, I remember getting up and saying "I did not like that one".

I kept picturing my cervix opening for the baby and each contraction getting my body more prepared to push her out. I do remember being tired, and feeling this night was so long, I wanted to take a break and finish it tomorrow after 8 hours of sleep. Jeff advised me to get up and walk, so I did. He walked me into the girls' room and pointed out the window to where the early light of morning was approaching….dawn. He said "look outside baby, do you see that…that is morning approaching, she is almost here. You will hold your baby before morning." Then *BAM*!!! The urge to push hit me; into the bathroom I ran and called out for Pamela, our Midwife. Jeff rushed to get Valkyrie who was stirring from my primal labor sounds that came from deep within. With the first push my water broke. There we were: the 5 of us crammed into this tiny hall bathroom. I gave literally 5 pushes and there she was…in my arms.

This beautiful tiny body, Skyler was here! She was a healthy 8 lbs 4oz and 20 ½ inches long. *I did it!* It was an amazing, wonderful birth. I never did get a chance to call our friends back over, it happened too fast. I sat there holding my baby girl for awhile, taking in this breathtaking moment. (The total labor was about 16 hours long).

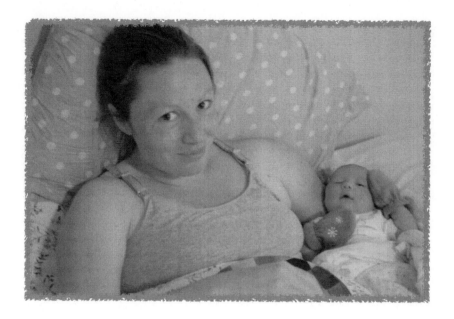

# My Journey Through Birth by Hue Anh

It was May of 2005 that I discovered I was pregnant with my daughter unexpectedly. It was only recently that I had a cystectomy of my ovary. I didn't anticipate having a baby any time soon. I felt lots of uncertainty, with the situation that I was in. A rocky marriage, a trauma to my body from a motor vehicle accident. In spite of all of that, this is a chance for me to have my dream birth, I realized.

I used kinesiology and tested for a positive result, then double checked it with an over the counter pregnancy test. I didn't really go in to get tested until I was 6 weeks. After watching my friend and also my birth attendant's unassisted birth video, I really enjoyed the calmness and the empowerment that went with the birth. They were so much in control and with so much peace at her birth.

I still went to my midwife for prenatal care. This time around I took care of my body really well despite all the discomfort I was experiencing with trauma caused by my previous car accident only months earlier. I already had planned for this birth to be at home, of which never happened with my first two births. This will be a dream come true. Ever since I had children I always wanted a home birth and didn't for various reasons. With all my positive experience with my pregnancy and eating well, healthy exercise, with all the health progress, it was surprising my hospital based midwife asked me if I ever thought of having a home-birth. I told her yes. I never told her I was planning it that way.

With her suggestion, I was comfortable to bring it up to my husband. However, I wasn't welcomed with the idea. Like 97% of the people out there, my husband and mother in law drowned me in all the safety issue, and negativity. So, since then I never spoke of it again. Between my birth attendant and I, we went ahead and planned out the birth. I started visualizing how wonderful, safe, calm and peaceful the birth was to be. Every day I would meditate and visualize.

My birth attendant had organized a wonderful Blessing Way for me with just women, and it was a very special day. Not so much commercial like the baby shower. I felt really special and pampered. The Blessing Way was friends coming together with flowers, candles and beads and gifts of choice for mummy to be and baby if they wished. And the sharing of *POSITIVE BIRTH STORIES* was highly suggested. Everyone had came up with the positive stories about their birth, and focusing on the positive aspect of the experience. I had a cast made of my 36 weeks belly. Even there, I was reluctant to share my birth wishes with anyone, except a couple of close, open minded and supportive friends.

Weeks prior, through planning with my birth attendant, I had purchased a nice kid pool big enough to soak in and easy to blow up. It was February when I was due. The weather that I imagined would be clear and nice blue sky. I bought liners from the home-birth place, and ordered tank heaters from the farmer's supplies online. I was able to heat up the birth tub and tried it out a couple of nights prior.

By this time, my husband is working out of town. I had two kids to take care of, so I had made plans with my neighbor who is also a wonderful friend for child care. Lucky for me, my husband was home late Thursday, days sooner than he was intended to come back. Friday morning came, it was 4:30 AM that I started feeling contractions. It was getting frequent, and I didn't want to disturb my husband, so I went downstairs and filled up my tub, getting the last pieces together. As the daylight came, the contractions got more frequent and intense. I decided to call my birth attendant and she made arrangements for her children. Two hours later she showed up on my door step and I was very calm with all the contractions I had experienced. I felt very quiet about it and the contractions became less frequent when my whole family woke up.

My attendant was helping to mend my bean bag and got everything laid out. I took out my colorful cord ties that I had made weeks prior and I started to light some candles from my Blessing Way. I wore my beautiful beaded necklace that was put together by my birth attendant from women friends that came or sent in by mail. I had soft, relaxing music and essential oils.

The contractions were getting more intense, so we sent the children off. At this time, my husband was working upstairs and kept asking me when am I going to the hospital?. 'Soon', I said. I had kept it to myself, since he wasn't supportive of the idea, and I do not want any more conflict and argument that it could lead to. So I had to let him believe that I am having a hospital birth.

Thankfully, the weather was nice and warm and dry as I had imagined all these months leading to the birth. So, my friend/attendant and I went for nature walk to the park. I spent an hour or so there, the contractions were getting intense. Every other step we took getting back to my house I would go down on my knees and wait until the contraction was over. We kept walking before hundreds of contractions had gone by, it seemed, and then we finally made it home. I felt I was ready for the hot tub and my attendant got more warm water. There I relaxed and labored. Thankfully, I was in water, as my hips weren't in the best shape due to my trauma from MVA. It was past 2 PM, and my neighbor called and I had the children back. So, my husband took care of them upstairs.

It was really intense labor for hours. I spent time meditating and really tuning into my body, where I wouldn't have been able to if I was in the hospital. No vital checks were made, no measuring of blood pressure or intervention needed to be done. I felt really empowered to be in tune with my own birth. The support was wonderful from my attendant. She was incredibly knowledgeable, (but the ancient kind of experience, not 'professional'). She knew when the moment had come and told me it will be my last potty visit if I want to do it now, so I did. The moment I stood up from the toilet, I felt my thigh was firming up, and all tensed up, my body was ready to deliver this baby.

So, we called my husband down, and from a distance, he took a video of the birth. I really knew when this baby was coming. I wasn't told when to push, my body knew exactly what to do. Before some more intense contraction, baby arrived asleep, the water was so warm and the birth was so peaceful, she had to be woken up. My baby was so beautiful, the pool was so clean, I was moved to my comfortable beanbag, where I held and nursed her. Soon after, I had given birth to the placenta. I was then able to cut the cord and tied it up with my colorful braided cord ties.

My birth was exactly how I had envisioned; the peace and joy with it, I was able to rest on my own bed after. She arrived after 3 PM, on a Friday, so I just let the hospital know that I had her, so I could later do some paper work. Baby was over 8 lbs, and I had a little tear, and didn't have much discomfort.

I couldn't have asked for more. This is the birth I had dreamt of, and would never do it any other way. I have so much to be thankful for, including a wonderful friend and birth attendant. I had my physical therapist over the next day, correcting my body and working on me. My massage therapist came the day after. This is heaven. I couldn't have done with out the wonderful home visit by my therapist and friend. My body wouldn't have recovered so quickly if I had gone any other route.

# Fantasy

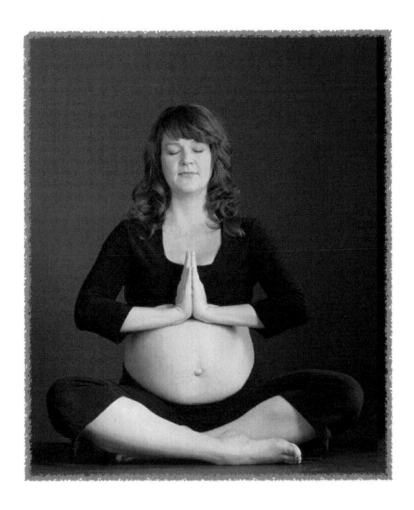

There is nothing more powerful in life than thoughts. In fact, thoughts are what mold who we are, how we function in life and what the world around us looks and operates like. Just to bring it in to the focus of pregnancy, imagine every day you woke up thinking about being sick, injured or miserable. It is certain that given a enough time, you will experience this. Like-wise, if you wake daily, thinking that the day will be amazing and fantastic, then it most likely will be, admitting that there are days that would naturally deviate. We've all read and heard how powerful thoughts are, but I tell you, it is your *Duty* to diligently guard your thoughts while pregnant!

There might never be a more fearful time for you than during pregnancy. There might be so many fears associated with pregnancy, labor, birth and mothering that you are paralyzed by it. This is where the deep need for attention to and care of your psychological state is imperative. The more fears that you have, the harder you should work at addressing and releasing these fears, because what we think about, we do manifest. This is a time to let go of those fears and trust that life and birth work. While I believe that birth is as safe as life gets, I do also recognize that there can be deviations from normal that are a cause for some level of fear. Fear at it's most fundamental level is healthy. It causes heightened senses and responses. This is to cause you to react and respond, aiding a positive result. However, when we live with fears day to day, it not only wears the mind and body down, it makes it more likely that we will live what we fear. Again, if you find you do have fears about pregnancy, labor and birth, I strongly encourage the book previously referred to by the name of, *Creating a Joyful Birth Experience* by Lucia Capacchione and Sandra Bardley.

To make this more clear, imagine that you are walking along a side walk and a car veers toward you. You are flooded with fear and hormones that cause you to re-act. You jump out of the way. This was an instance when fear was good. However, also imagine that you are pregnant and fear that you will end up with a cesarean. Each day your body functions with a subtle, but present undercurrent of stress hormones that eventually impact your health in some way and also bring about that which you fear.

So, now that most people will, in fact, accept the fact that our thoughts form our reality, let's do something with that! Let's let ourselves use our mind as a tool and treat yourself to fantasy. Fantasy can be one of the most powerful exercises that you can do while pregnant. Actually, if a person could choose only one great thing to do for themselves during pregnancy, I would say that this should be it. I found that when I took time fantasizing about labor and birth, I would be able to bring about an almost high feeling of euphoria. These hormones flood the body and even baby, and are highly nurturing.

There are some important rules to apply to birth fantasies and they are that they are positive, free from complications and that they can be in any setting with no limits of what is 'reality'. Meaning, if you want to fantasize about laboring in the ocean, then do it. There should be no limit to what is possible. This doesn't mean that you are really going to go labor in the ocean, although that too, is a possibility. The idea is that you fantasize about your labor and birth and create the birth of your dreams in this fantasy. The mind is powerful. As you draw closer to the birth, you may find that you get a little more real with your fantasy, bringing it in to your chosen birth environment, but that is no reason to make it less enjoyable.

Daily, while you rest and more frequently, if possible, spend at least 15 minutes fantasizing about your dream labor and birth.

# My Journey Through Birth by Brandi:

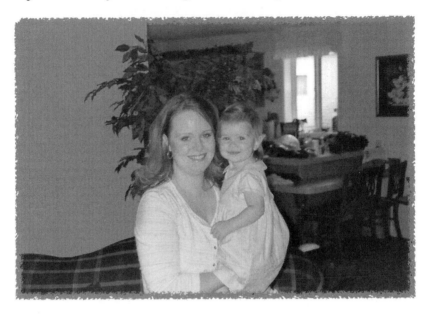

It's fitting that since birth is a journey for the baby, I too had a progressive journey with my three birth stories.

My first story, from my view, was uneducated. My husband and I did everything by the book when we were supposed to do it. Doctor appointments, blood tests, exams, ultra sounds, even an amniocentesis. The doctor always had the "right" answers, so why did we need to go elsewhere for them? I would discover the reasons and real answers through my next two births. So, of course as soon as my water broke (on my due date) we made our way to the hospital with excitement and anticipation of meeting our new little boy.

I continued to labor for 17 hours with very little progress. I did most of my laboring on my back in a hospital bed hooked up to monitors. There was no "hands on" from the nurses or doctor, but since my cervix wasn't dilating past four centimeters, it was decided to give me Pitocin and Stadol. Several hours later, that still wasn't working, and I was so tired and in so much pain from the Pitocin, I decided to have an epidural. Just as the anesthesiologist was about to administer it, my doctor came in and stopped him. He said it was time for a cesarean. Period. That's what the doctor said and I was sure he knew best. After all, this was his job, right? So, after 17 hours we met our sweet boy via cesarean.

I was struck by the pain and inability to move after my surgery. I remember thinking back to our childbirth education classes we took at the hospital and never once could I recall the instructor teaching about the recovery of a cesarean. I was in for a shock. I couldn't understand why my body did not birth a five pound 15 ounce baby. I do freshly recall my doctor joking that I better have the baby by 7 PM, because that's when he was supposed to watch his pay per view of the Tyson/Holyfield fight (remember the one when Tyson bit Holyfield's ear?)! You bet, our son came by cesarean before that. Our son was born at 4:40 PM.

At my post-op appointment my doctor told me our son's head was too big to fit through my pelvis and that my pelvis was too small to birth a baby any bigger than my son. At the time I accepted that statement as truth. It must have been true since I couldn't even birth a five pound baby, right? I would later find out from my operative report that our son was posterior. Never once was that mentioned throughout my labor. I don't even believe the nurses or doctor knew that because they never felt for it or tried to correct the baby's position nor was it stated in my preoperative diagnosis.

I knew I wanted things to be different when I learned I was pregnant the second time. I started seeing a certified nurse midwife in a nearby town at the recommendation of my new childbirth educator (who would become my best girlfriend). I began the healing process of my cesarean and started reading recommended books. My favorite book being Immaculate Deception by Suzanne Arms. My husband and I took childbirth education classes in our home with a few other couples and I felt focused and capable. I believed I could have a VBAC (vaginal birth after cesarean). I felt I had made progress as far as making more of my own decisions about my pregnancy and birth, but still put much trust in my midwife. I loved the fact that she would be an advocate for a safe and natural birth and she truly believed I could have a VBAC. Once again I began labor by my water breaking (on my due date, again!). It seemed like déjà vu.

I called my best friend and she was over soon after. I labored at home for five hours, but was scared because I was bleeding some, so we drove to the hospital. I tried walking, laboring in a birthing pool in my room and also labored on the bed. I loved that I wasn't confined to my bed like last time. After eleven hours I decided to have an epidural. I really didn't want the drugs, but I was ready for some relief. I felt very uptight and tired at the length of my labor so far and therefore my body was reacting to that and not progressing. At this point there was some concern that if I didn't start dilating more I would have to have another cesarean. After the epidural, I was able to relax and even get a little rest. So after a total of 17 hours, we had a successful VBAC and I was holding another sweet boy! And I was most excited because he was 7 pounds 6 ounces. I could birth a baby the way God created my body to do it! I felt empowered and had learned so much about my body through this pregnancy, but didn't realize how much more I needed to learn for my next birth.

I was witnessing something amazing: my best friend's unassisted water birth. After the beautiful birth of her baby girl her husband asked me if I was ready for a home birth. I quickly said no way! I didn't know it at the time, but I was pregnant and I would have a home birth. At my first appointment with my midwife I was very upset to find out that all the nearby hospitals had, by law, put a ban on VBACs. This was to prevent doctors from malpractice lawsuits due to VBACs supposedly being at a higher risk for uterine ruptures. I was crushed since I had already had a VBAC. I knew I could do it again. So began the biggest mental, emotional and physical growth process I had ever had. I found a home birth midwife and assistant that I felt very comfortable with and began reading anything I could find about home births. I did prenatal yoga, stretching and a lot of visualization. I also created a positive affirmation tape all about my birth and how I wanted it to be with Enya playing in the background. I listened to the tape every night when I went to bed while I practiced breathing and relaxation techniques. I felt like I couldn't have prepared any better. I truly believed I was doing the best thing I could do for me and my baby.

I'm known as a jokester, so when I called my best friend at 10 PM on April Fools and told her my water broke she thought I was kidding. I felt like everything I had learned momentarily left my brain and all I could think of was this is how my other births started. My girlfriend prayed for me and gently reminded me this birth would be different. Was she ever right. I called my midwife and she advised me to try to get some rest, it could be a while. When I couldn't rest because the contractions were coming every couple minutes I called her back and had a contraction while on the phone. She then very quickly said she would be at my house right away. She arrived about 30 minutes later. Her assistant lived about 45 minutes away, but she would be leaving soon.

I remember feeling so calm throughout the labor, even when my midwife told me we needed to turn the baby slightly. I used an exercise ball to roll on and the baby turned. As soon as that happened things moved very quickly. So quickly, in fact, my best friend and midwife's assistant arrived only minutes before the birth. All my hard work of educating myself had paid off and the prize was a sweet little angel girl! (Of course born on her due date!) The two boys slept soundly through the birth in the room right next to us. They woke up and held their little sister just moments after she was born. I believe this four hour labor and delivery vs. the previous 17 hour labors was due to me trusting my body to do what it was supposed to do. At that point I would have loved to have more babies just for the home birth experience! I'm convinced my first two births would have been quicker and less painful had I known all I do now. My favorite part of the experience was cuddling with our new little girl in our own bed later that morning. I feel so blessed to have had the people in my life that encouraged me along the way and for our home birth to be such an awesome experience.

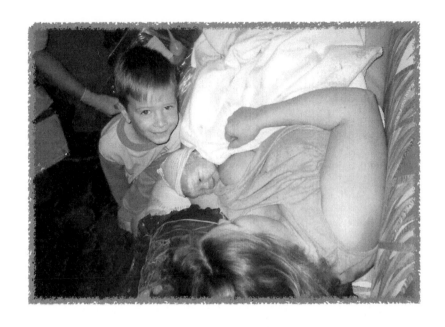

## Creation

Blood pulses, body releases. Life flows, mobility decreases. Belly expands, normality ceases. Breasts blossom, creation surges. Fluid suspends, continuum urges. Life cycles, identity purges.

by Tara L. McGuire

~~~~~~~~~~~~~~~~~~~~~~~~~

## Kara's Birth

WRITHING, TWISTING yearning to be free I feel you move
inside of me I spread, I Open, I am ESTATIC
MY eager hands await your emergence
Your head pops out, like a little groundhog I push quick and fast
and your shoulders slip through
your momentum carries you into my fingers Then I sweep you up
into my thankful arms I LOVE YOU BABY, I whisper, elated.
I kiss your wet head, and snuggle you to my chest. So glad you are
home at last.

by Danielle Saxon

# My Journey Through Birth by Sarah

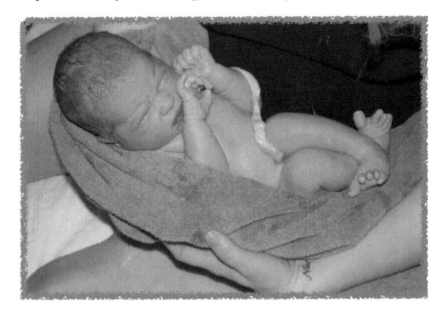

February 19, 2010 I woke up with a contraction and it quickly drove me out of bed. I'd been having them for several weeks and didn't notice anything different with this one. I laid back down only to have another one follow, so I got up to start the day. It had been a hard few months so I was very grateful for such a smooth pregnancy. We'd moved to a new house on my due date and nine days later I had brought order to the place... mostly. I spent the time before my husband and daughter woke up finding places for odds and ends around the house. It felt good here. We were out in the country on 5 acres, the house was roomy. I didn't know in the beginning where I would give birth but now standing in the kitchen looking out on the snow covered pines, it all felt like it finally fit.

I knew labor would begin soon. I was dilated to about 4cm and had lost my mucous plug the previous day. Many women in our culture view the end of pregnancy with urgency, a need to escape the less than comfortable physical state and "get it over with." After giving birth to my first child at 35 weeks this was a completely different journey than the first time and I was not at all anxious for it to end. I knew that pregnancy was the easy part and as we had decided this was to be our last child I was not quite ready to let go of the experience. Now everything was in order, it was only my husband and I and our emotions stalling the process.

I cooked breakfast for my husband and 2 year old daughter and sent them out into the snowy world. I needed my space this morning. I cranked up my music and sang my heart out as I washed dishes and cleaned, fighting to reach a place of readiness and transition for what was coming. At 11 o'clock I realized I couldn't hide the contractions from anyone if they saw me. This must be it. I drove to a prenatal visit with a midwife at a friend's house at about 1 PM.

I desperately wanted to hide my labor from the midwife. I had wanted an unassisted birth all along but felt somewhat obligated to have a midwife. My husband thought I had lost it when I talked about a drug free birth after finding out I was pregnant with our second child. Compromise was reached when I employed a certified professional midwife from a neighboring state. I did not mesh with her at all and dreaded the thought of actually having her present at my most vulnerable moments. After all my efforts to inundate Nick with information he started joking about doing it ourselves around 37 weeks. I just resolved to let labor decide.

My contractions stopped when I stepped foot out of the car and didn't return until I reached home again. I was worried it had stopped altogether. Nick and Adison were napping when I got home and I tried to lay down with them but an intense contraction propelled me right back up out of bed. Still not convinced my labor had resumed I took a warm bath and drank a glass of wine. I couldn't sit long enough to enjoy it and it didn't slow things down a bit.

When I had to work through contractions on all fours I realized it was time for my daughter to leave. She was on all fours mimicking me but it also seemed to frighten her a bit even though I was not yet vocalizing. It felt like a long hour taking care of her waiting for my mom to arrive to pick her up at 6 PM.

I spent a lot of time on all fours on the stairs and began vocalizing about 8 PM. I had been listening to Hypnobabies all day but it felt so good to release the energy of the contraction through vocalization. I judged myself to be around 8 or 9 cm dilated and slipping in and out of transition. Nick wanted to go to the gym and I didn't want to be alone in the house but told him to go anyway. Thankfully he turned the truck around and came back. While he supported me in a drug free birth it also brought him to a great feeling of helplessness so we agreed that as long as he was physically present that was all I needed. He was watching a movie on his computer and had his headphones on. I was on my knees leaning on our double rocking chair, rocking my way through contraction after contraction.

I was having intense back and thigh labor. Upright positions were all I could tolerate. I couldn't even sit on the toilet without incredible cramping in my periformus muscle. Nick tried pushing on my back and squeezing my hips but it didn't take the edge off. I was getting frustrated with the cervical lip and contemplating calling the midwife. Stuck in transition is not an easy place to be. I went to the basement to take a shower at about 10:30 PM hoping to relax enough to finish dilating. I was very tired. I put my arms on the bars in the shower and rested my head falling asleep standing up between contractions. They were two minutes apart at this point.

The hot water lasted about an hour and made me wish that I had ordered a birthing tub. It took enough of the edge off that I felt very clear headed for the first time in a while. I was very aware

131

of my body as I contemplated my options. Should I call the midwife to help me through the cervical lip? Should I try pushing past it? I knew that I could risk tearing my cervix or cause it to swell so much that a cesarean would end up my only option. As the hot water ran out I felt resolved to continue on my own.

I asked Nick if he had any qualms about continuing on our own. I felt completely confident and peaceful about our decision. I knelt over a chux pad in our plastic wrapped living room and checked myself again. No change. The bag of waters was well past my cervix and I decided to break it. I knew it might take things to the next level and was I ever right. Within two contractions I was fully dilated. They came harder then; the jump in intensity level took my breath away. Vocalizing was not enough, I fought with all I had to keep my body relaxed but it was insanely difficult. I was strangely lucid between rushes but each one whisked me away to far off labor land.

I moved around quite a bit waiting for the urge to push. Nick told me that I should rest so I tried laying on the couch. It was so easy to slip off to sleep in the minute between them but they brought me roaring back with ferocity. It started getting hard to breathe; I felt like I was going to hyperventilate. At that point I begged Nick to talk me through breathing with each contraction. I felt like I was in a vice grip and inhaling took all my concentration. I moved back to my favorite position of kneeling in front of the rocking chair and tried pushing on my own.

I had had an overwhelming urge to push during my first birth. It had been the worst feeling to not push when I wanted to. Finally after pushing through a few contractions the urge came out of nowhere. I'm not sure how long I was pushing. I realized I must not have been communicating very well earlier because my husband thought we had all night to go yet and was shocked by my telling him that her head was in the birth canal. I gave him a review between contractions. What to check for first, what was normal and what was not. I was amazed at how all consuming the pushing was yet how clear headed I felt between rushes. He disappeared then and told me later he was grabbing last minute items and closing the vents in the rest of the house so the living room would be warm. It still makes me laugh that he didn't realize how near the end it all was.

I felt her crowning and held her back with a cloth covered in olive oil. Nick said I was talking to her, telling her to slow down but I don't remember. I know I literally held her in through 3 contractions, I was so scared of tearing and she was much bigger than my first baby. Nick kept telling me to push her out and I kept saying I wasn't ready. Then it felt right so I moved my hand and pushed with all my might. It felt very strange, not like I had expected or remembered. Instead of feeling relief after her head was out it felt more intense as I felt her shoulders and hips pass out of me. I found out later that she was facing the correct direction but had her right hand against her forehead and her left shoulder was up by her ear. Her hand did not extend so I had the width of her shoulder, head and elbow to contend with. Her whole body came out in a massive push that made me vomit a little.

I heard the excitement in his voice, "She has so much hair!" I turned around and sat down on the chux pads anxious to see the little person making such a loud fuss. As I pulled her to my chest Nick put a warm towel around her and she peed on me! My friends said it was because she looked around and saw there was no midwife present. Chevelle Liberty was born at 1:20 AM on February 20th, after 14 hours of labor.

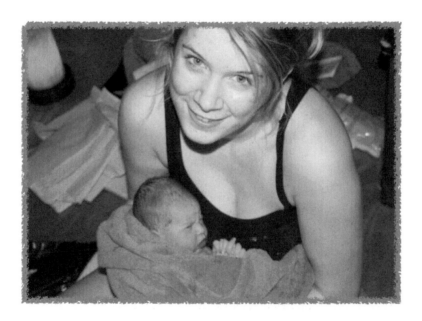

She stopped crying as I held her and I gazed in awe of the perfect little being in my arms. Her head had no molding and her coloring was so perfect. She was so big! After having a 35 weeker she seemed like a 3 month old! She didn't need any suction and very little clean up. I was shocked at how clean the whole ordeal was. I only used 2 chux pads through the labor and only lost a few tablespoons of blood. She wasn't interested in nursing so I just held her. Her cord stopped pulsing and we cut it about 20 minutes after she was born. Then the after pains began. They were no less intense than before and I had to vocalize through them. I couldn't hold her when one hit, so Nick got her dressed and held her. Soon I realized it'd been 45 minutes and she hadn't nursed yet so I took her and laid down in bed. She did nurse a bit and then went to sleep.

It was a wonderful feeling to be snug in my own bed so soon after delivery. I was absolutely in love with the alert, smiling newborn I already felt such a connection with. The contractions continued but my placenta didn't come. I set up everything I'd need beside the bed and tried to rest waiting for it. The after pains felt so much more intense when I just wanted to sleep. I wanted to be done! I pulled lightly on the cord but to no avail. Exactly 2 hours after birth it came out all in one piece. There was quite a bit of blood and fluid with it and I watched very carefully for signs of hemorrhage as it had occurred during my first birth. I went through 3 pads immediately and visualized turning off a faucet in my uterus. The bleeding slowed considerably and I made myself a sandwich and drank some juice. At last, I drifted off to sleep, cherub in arms.

The next day the midwife came with her assistants to check out the baby. She knew that I might not call her and had made it clear she was unsupportive. She herself had had an unassisted birth and it was strange to me that she was so opposed to it. Looking back I wish I hadn't called her at all but just taken the baby to see my back up obstetrician instead. She was a buzz kill with her attitude. The one good thing that came from her visit was being able to weigh Chevelle. She was 7 lbs 4 oz. She also confirmed that I had no tears, just one skid mark.

We hadn't told anyone of our plans to go it alone and I especially was worried about people's reactions. I might have kept it private and said we'd had a midwife but Nick beat me to sharing the news and he wasn't about to downplay his importance as Dr. Dad. He certainly deserved the credit as I couldn't have done it without him at the end. His take it or leave it attitude has helped me feel even more empowered by Chevelle's birth.

I have been so impressed by the difference letting nature take its course can make. I didn't experience detachment like I did after an epidural. I haven't struggled in the slightest with postpartum depression while I suffered horribly with it with my first child. Breastfeeding came much more naturally and I've been able to stick with it. I had difficulty bonding with my first child but that has not been so this time around. This birth has been very healing for me, not only healing of my first birth which I felt was traumatic and full of needless interventions but also healing of childhood incest. It is easy to know in your head that sexuality is not your body's only purpose but it was a beautiful experience during labor to be able to realize, this is what my body is made for and it is valuable and momentous.

The difficulty level and length of my labor was not something I fully anticipated, I had spent a great deal of time visualizing a quick, pain free birth. I think that the way it went was what I truly needed though. It gave me time to work through things mentally and really enjoy the experience, even if it wasn't pain free. It has deepened my sense of inner strength that I will have to draw on for the rest of my life.

**Affirmations for a joyful pregnancy and birth:**

I breathe in peace and exhale, surrendering.

My body is strong, open and ready to release my child and I eagerly embrace this journey.

My mind is calm and full of love, light and trust.

My body and my baby are beautifully built for birth.

With patience, trust and intuition, I lovingly open to the work of birth.

Each day, I embrace the changes in my growing body and each day, I cherish the time that I have with my unborn baby.

(Your name), I love you and thank you for exactly who and where you are right now.

Everything that I need to labor and birth my baby safely is already within me.

Daily, I quiet myself to hear the small

# Intervention

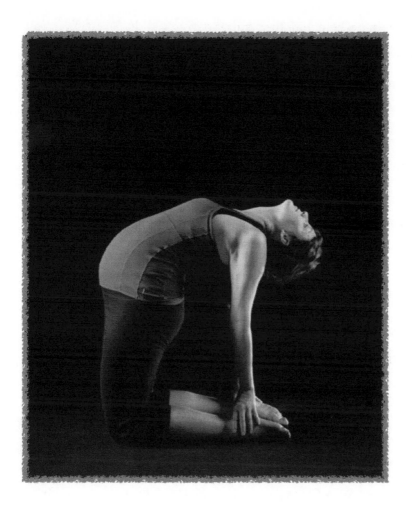

I would hope that by this point, you have understood that I would like to communicate the respect for intervention when appropriately applied. I believe in unassisted birth and free birth and I also believe in the presence of an attendant. Some women will not want the responsibility of outcome to lie on them. Having a birth attendant, to a large extent, transfers that responsibility to the attendant in a woman's eyes, be it midwife or doctor. I have heard stories where a mother and or baby lived due to intervention and I have heard stories where a mother and or baby died due to intervention and I have likewise heard of the stories where one or both did die despite the presence or absence of intervention.

Without being flippant about the value of life, I will state that birth happens and death happens. They are both a part of life and there are times when the two meet and it is beyond devastating. A woman (and her man if present), need to face and own the fact that these are truths regardless of whether they choose to have an attendant or not. A woman need to own the fact that this is her body and her baby and that she is the one to be responsible for the interventions, if any, that will be applied during her pregnancy, labor, birth, and postpartum. Simply allowing a doctor or midwife to make decisions for you when you are capable of making those decisions is lazy. There are times when you will obviously consider the input of the professional that you have chosen, but make no mistake; the choice is yours. The result is then your choice.

I've seen too many women and couples placing their trust and care solely in the hands of their chosen professional and then turn around and be disappointed in the results. They often then go through a process of empowerment and this can take several births to get to the point that they feel that they had the result of truly owning their pregnancy and birth. This does not, however, imply that deviations from 'normal' are not part of that process.

There can be intervention in an unassisted, or unattended birth. There can be intervention in a midwife attended birth and there can be intervention in a doctor attended birth. When utilized as a response to a deviation to the normal physiological process, it can be helpful, but when used as a course in the normal 'management' of pregnancy, labor and birth, it is harmful and damaging. This medicalization of childbirth is an archaic approach; one who's time has come to an end, as more an more birthing families choose empowerment over weakness and pro-activeness over non-involvement in the process and choices we face in the birthing of our babies.

While I whole-heartedly know and affirm that a woman and baby are safer birthing at home, I too believe that a woman will birth best where she feels safest. I do not condemn a woman for her choice of birth location. I do know that numbers don't lie and she is much more likely to have a cesarean in a hospital and she is much less likely to have a satisfying birth experience out of her home.

However, with more education, a woman who does not feel safe at home, will likely be able to trust and know that she is, in fact, safer at home. So, either a woman empower herself and educate herself to that point, or she ought to expend the effort and energy to create a safe birth in the hospital. I simply believe that it takes much more effort and energy to create a safe, natural birth in a hospital environment than it is worth. There is always the middle road choice of a birth center which can ease some of the fears surrounding birth, but I really would rather address those fears and let the low risk and average mother birth in the home, where the child was likely created and in a like-setting as well.

The tools necessary in a birth ought to be the ones used for love-making. Some candles, soft music, and if you are so inclined, a bottle of wine. The same hormones that get the baby in, get the baby out.

Midwifery Today:

The past several decades of obstetrics has also taught us how to save lives. Midwives can blend the wise and restrained use of technology with good midwifery education and be prepared to meet just about any challenge that may present itself in a woman's pregnancy or birth. Midwives then tailor their care to the individual's own needs and beliefs. They take responsibility for educating clients about their choices and for making these choices as available as possible.

Midwifery Today PO Box 2672 Eugene, OR 97402 USA

*"...normal birth is what is normal for a particular woman. There are no rigorous time frames that say a woman "should" do something at a given time. Each woman and baby unit finds their own way to birth. It's a long process for some and shorter for others. If the mother and baby are doing well, there is no need to intervene with an expectation of time. Left to her own devices, with warmth and support, women birth most easily on their own. Medicalized births happen because of the belief that all women's bodies function the same way. This is like saying that all women get turned on or have orgasms from the same things or positions. Nothing could be farther from the truth. Western medicine*

*views our bodies in a very linear fashion: that a "normal" menstrual cycle is 28 days and that all women "normally" ovulate on day 14. That all "normal" pregnancies are 40 weeks long. It's this type of thinking that leaves women feeling like their bodies failed them ("I couldn't dilate", "I couldn't make enough milk", "I cannot start labor on my own"), when, in fact, it is the system that fails their bodies." Pamela Hines-Powel CPM.*

# My Journey Through Birth by Amy:

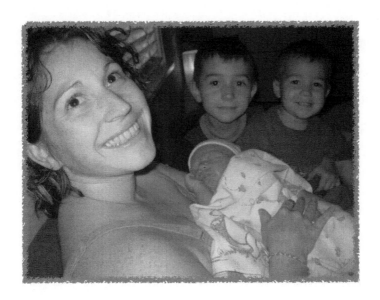

*My birth history:*

*1994: Vaginal Hospital Delivery (horrible experience)*

*1997: Surrogate Pregnancy/Delivery Twins, breech, c-section*

*1999: Repeat C-section at dr's request 2 week early baby (NICU for 5 days)*

*2002: First VBAC/ Hospital, AROM, Pit, Epidural, and vag. Delivery*

*2003: Miscarriage that changed our lives, and view of labor, birth, etc.*

*2004: Unassisted Pregnancy: Midwife hired at the end 2 weeks before home waterbirth. Baby born 3 weeks early.*

*2006: Completely Unassisted Pregnancy and Birth*

*2009: Mostly Unassisted Pregnancy and Midwife and family attended home water-birth.*

September 29, 2006 Friday 10:45 AM, I am 39-40 weeks. I have so many things I'd like to do, but I am just so tired, and achey. I think the aches and pains, and the emotional side of things is what is getting the better of me. I read yesterday about the possibility of our baby not being in an optimal position. It seems like he is lying on my left side most days, although I don't think he's posterior. Under my ribs on my right side still is so tight and painful, especially while sitting up. I don't have hardly a sign of labor as far as I can tell. No mucous, hardly any contractions, no diarrhea, no frequent peeing, and so on.

I tried doing the positions recommended to get him in the LOA, left side of my body, last night, from an online book I read. Leaning over pillows on an ottoman while we all watched a family movie. And last night I stayed on my left side, with the belly down low, a pillow between my legs. I didn't lay on my back or right side, and my back started getting awful pains in the middle of the night.

The book I read said that was normal until the baby shifts sides, and to stay that way. I am just so tired and sore. It was a difficult night. Every time I got up it was a reminder that I may not be any where close to delivery, and I just want to cry most of the time.

I am so thankful for Eddie's support, and for the encouragement, but I really feel like I've been ready to birth for weeks now. I had believed it would be a September baby from the beginning of this pregnancy, and tomorrow is the last day of September. I obviously have no control over that, and I'm staying away from manipulating my body to trigger unnatural labor. If the contractions picked up but spaced off, I'd do nipple stimulation, and maybe walking around the block. We gave up on cervical checks now, as the last time Eddie could barely find it.

The other children are handling things very well, and I'm sure they have appreciated the time Eddie has been able to give to all of us through this.

I just don't know what to do, or if I'm doing something to keep labor from starting. I don't want to be the reason the baby isn't engaging. I am tired, and I just feel like laying down most of the time. I will try to stay on my left side all day today, despite the sore back muscles. Maybe I will feel some engagement later. I will update more later.

October 9, 2006 Monday 5:10 AM. Well, according to my lmp, a doctor would consider today my due date. I honestly didn't think today would arrive and I would be sitting at the computer, very pregnant.

I was laying in bed going over some thoughts, and some interesting thoughts came to mind. The first being: I feel *VERY* past-due! There is an absolute truth that should chase away discouragement. The truth that God began this work and He will see it completed in me. I don't need to doubt the 'whys' of my circumstances. I don't need to question God's will and timing.

You see, when 'real' labor starts, nothing can stop it. All these different days where I've had false labor attempts, where I prepared to birth and then it stopped; I never stopped and questioned God's will for our baby to be born. It wasn't a matter of if our baby would birth, it's always been a matter of when..and that is ultimately up to God. That has really helped me this morning.

So, the challenges of this weekend have been wondering if baby is doing ok, and what his position is. Is there more I can do to help him engage? I had a friend attempt a UC last week, and she transferred after pushing for 3 hours. Turns out, her little guy wasn't so little, 11 lbs. 4oz and 22 ½ inches long. She is healthy and so is he, but she's never had to deliver any of her other 3 bio children in a hospital. It clearly has shaken her up a bit. I'm so thankful that she and her son are healthy and safe, and she didn't have to have a c-section.

The changes in my body and pregnancy are….I have most certainly gained close to 70 lbs.. I have days where I have contractions that last hours, sometimes all day, but as soon as bedtime they go away. I will then have a day of *NO* contractions and not a lot of movement from baby boy (we have now picked the name Elias). The movements I do get from him now are not very active or that big. Some rolls and stretching, but it's rare that I get a BIG active spurt out of him. I got more activity from him last night after about 7 PM, it causes some pressure down low, but no contractions came with his activity. I just stayed hands off of interventions yesterday. No cohoshes. Eddie tried to check for dilation once again, but just had the hardest time reaching my cervix. It feels like Elias is head down, but we just don't know for sure. He switches from left side to right side.

My ribs barely hurt now. In fact, I don't have any rib discomfort the whole time I've been sitting here typing. I am sweating A *LOT* at night. I'm not sure what that is, but I'm assuming it's hormonal. I don't sleep in anything but underwear and wake up with freezing arms, but everything else is sweaty. It's a little frustrating. I will lose a little clear/yellowish mucous every now and then, but nothing that has the least amount of blood in it. Still no signs of diarrhea.

Contractions aren't painful, and don't seem to last very long when I get them now. I don't have to pee constantly like I guess I should be expecting for being due. The only time I wake up to pee is when I get a contraction that wakes me a bit and makes me feel like I need to go. If I don't get up to pee after the contraction, the need to pee goes away, and I could fall asleep until another contraction wakes me up, but I usually just decide to get up and go. When I roll from my left side (which I am sleeping on regularly now, not my right side at all) to my back I always get a big contraction. Really, any big change in my position causes one, but they are just too small.

The strangest part to me this morning, is that I had days in September where I was certain birth was so close. Where I was certain that by the next day, Elias would be here. Now, I sit here, and I don't feel any of that. It feels like I'm uncomfortable, and that there just hasn't been any progress at all. I *KNOW* that isn't the truth, but that's how it feels to sit here. I don't feel much of anything right now. No real baby movements, no contractions, no rib pain, no pressure in my cervix. I am just sitting here very BIG. Eddie will probably be getting up soon, so I will end this in a minute.

Yesterday, Elias' heart rate kept changing on us (we rented a Doppler). We listened, and it would slow down and then speed up. I was worried because I think it got down to 130 bpm, and I'm not sure how fast it got. I don't know if contractions affected the heart rate for sure, but it was definitely a thought. We discussed the possibility of cord around his neck, but it just seems so much is out of our hands. We can't force labor to start, and we really don't want to go into the hospital to get their opinion on it, and let them decide how labor should go. Be it induction, water bag breaking, or worse, surgery. All of those things are very real possibilities if we go into the hospital.

We pray. We pray Elias is healthy and strong. We pray that the birth is amazing, and that both Elias and myself do wonderful through it, and heal quickly from it. That we are safe and that being at home, with just the privacy of our family, is what God wants from us. And should He want ours plans to change, may He reveal it to us, and guide us by His Spirit.

## *The Birth of Elias:*

October 9th at 11:08 PM. 9 lbs. 2oz and 22" long.
Believe it or not the rest of day progressed just as every other day. The sweet boy inside me barely moved (which concerned me) I would pray for peace. I had tried to tell if Elias was in an optimal position for weeks. It was so hard to tell. I have had one posterior that I know for sure, and suspect another one was, looking back at my past pregnancies. I was having a feeling that I should try squatting, but I had read and was told by my last midwife that it isn't a good idea if your baby is posterior. If he hadn't engaged posterior there was still a chance for him to turn, but if I did squats

I could engage him that way. Well, during the later part of the afternoon I decided to try. I squatted for as long as it was comfortable. I felt a little different upon standing up, but figured it was just muscles stretched. Had no real contractions or any others signs of impending labor.

Eddie came home from work and I tried squatting again. At 6:22 PM I wrote in my journal that I felt Elias move a little after eating dinner, and I was off to take a shower. I would try more squats after my shower. Well, getting ready for my shower I felt a contraction that only wrapped around the lower half of my abdomen, not at all up high like they'd been. It was tight, it was different, and my heart sped up. I *KNEW*, something inside told me with that first small, almost painless, but *DIFFERENT* contraction, that this was it. I went in to tell my husband and ask if he thought he should put just cold water in the pool incase this was the beginning. I was worried that things may go quickly if this was the beginning of labor, as I think I'd been laboring for weeks. I know I had already started dilating. He seemed skeptical..too many false starts I guess. And these didn't hurt, I was breathing through them, and here I was getting ready to shower and trying to tell him that I thought I was in labor finally. So I went to shower and the contractions continued down low, painless, but I could tell they were getting closer together. Dried my hair, got dressed comfortable, kids put to bed to read and relax.

At 7:30 PM, I told Eddie I not only wanted water in the pool, I strongly suggested that it be warm. He jumped up and came to feel the contractions with me. First one he felt, the next one 12 min. apart from that one. Ok, not very close. We excitedly got supplies laid out, pool started filling at 7:50 PM. We timed the contraction next one bigger and 9 min. The one after that was at 8:04 PM, now 5 min apart. By 9 PM, I was in the pool. The contractions spaced out and worried me, but the pain was enough that I knew I was in labor. I knew it was a matter of time and Elias would be with us finally.

I started worrying about the length of my labor after an hour. I have *NEVER* had my waters break naturally, and I was told that my last labor stalled, and wouldn't have progressed without the AROM or induction. We prayed through these fears time and time again. I finally decided to reach in and check. I felt what can be described at a small water balloon, not very filled up, and rubbery. I squeezed around it a little and didn't really feel anything in it. I instantly wondered if there was a foot coming out. Elias had been breech for so long, and we just prayed that he was head down. Either way, he was going to be born at home, but we wanted to do the best to prepare. I mentioned this concern to my Eddie, but he was excited and so funny through everything he never even thought twice about any of it. If it was breech, so be it, if it was a head, so be it. He was just so excited to be a part of this, and for it to be the two of us. All the children had fallen asleep, and we had music playing, candles lit, and we were enjoying being so close.

I drank my red raspberry leaf tea, between glasses of Emergan-C and ice water. Then the contractions changed and I got a little shaky. This took me by surprise because I hadn't felt this in labor before. I felt some pressure and decided to reach inside and see if there were changes and I felt pushy so I gave a little push while I felt the little bag of water come out a little bit more. When the contraction was over the little bag went back up a bit. Still no head or anything hard.

Ok, so now is where I do what I *ALWAYS* do in labor towards the end. Embarrassing, but I must admit it…I worry about having to pooh. I had a huge dinner that evening, not thinking I'd be delivering later, and I hadn't had any diarrhea. I was worried it would come out in the pool at some point while I was doing those little pushes. I wanted to stay in the pool (CLEAN) as long as possible. I knew with my phobia, that I would either hesitate to push all the way, or would push, mess up the pool and get out of the water where I was doing the best with the pain. I had told Eddie earlier that I didn't want to birth in the pool because I had a feeling that this baby needed to come out on land, but I changed my mind when I stood up from the pool and felt the difference between a contraction *IN* water and a contraction *OUT* of water. I told him that he would never get me out.

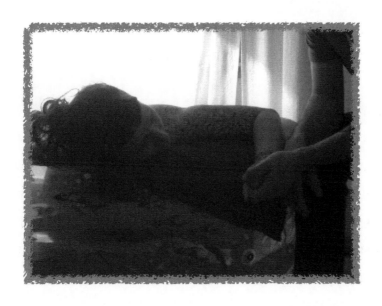

So, at some point between the more painful, shaky contractions, and starting to get a little pushy..I thought *THIS* would be a good time to run to my potty and see if I could pooh before delivery. We saw humor in this act almost immediately. I ran to the bathroom, Eddie followed, and I sat to squat..contraction hit, I pushed (what I thought would be my last pooh) and we heard a loud BANG and something fell (actually shot) into the potty. I stood up immediately and wondered, honestly, what had happened. Saw blood, but nothing else in the potty. Then the BIGGEST contraction of my life hit, my hubby dropped to his knees, don't know how he fit between the potty and tub, and I screamed like I've never screamed before. Instant pressure and something started to come out of me. We were in such shock. I locked my legs and couldn't move. I was standing over hubby and he kept saying I was doing a good job, just to keep breathing.

As I was screaming, I reached down and felt a *HUGE* round something come out. I instantly asked if it was a bottom. It was so big, much bigger than my last baby and didn't feel anything like a head. I kept trying to pant and breathe as it just stayed hanging out of me. The contraction was over, and I didn't believe Eddie when he said it was a head. He was half laughing. I yelled at him, and said, "then why isn't it crying?" He just chuckled again, and said to breathe and wait for the next contraction. I still heard no cries, and seriously thought he was fibbing to me to keep me calm, so I felt again. It just didn't feel like a head..*TOO BIG*. Eddie was so calm, he said "you're doing great, it's a head, now just breathe and wait for the next contraction."

Looking back, I'm so thankful to God that He led me to the bathroom for a land delivery after all. Had Elias been under water all this time, it would have really stressed me out. My contractions were spaced out, and then I asked if Eddie saw a cord around the neck. He said no, just as a contraction hit finally.

I screamed louder than before, and the body started to come out. Not too fast, and into hubby's hands. I looked down and saw what seemed to be a huge newborn laying on it's side. Hubby handed him to me, and instantly arrived with towels he'd been warming in the oven. I didn't even know he'd been so prepared. I was sitting on the potty holding our son, who had let out a beautiful *LOUD* scream when his body slipped out. His body was pink and looked so good. He was covered in thick vernix, especially on his head. It was very painful to push him out standing up like that, and I wouldn't choose that birth position ever again, but I do know in my heart, it's just what was needed for this birth.

For the labor and birth itself, it was the most remarkable experience of my life to date. God is so gracious, and all the glory is to Him for my strength and peace that He alone provided. My hubby was so patient and having the intimacy of the two of us was the most beautiful experience.

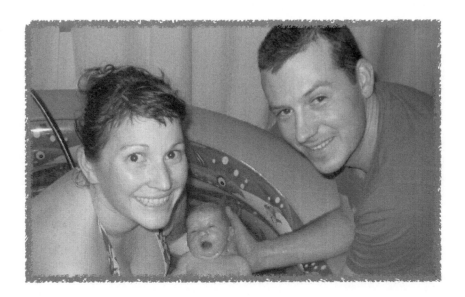

I am so thankful that we have in our arms a healthy and beautiful baby boy. I am thankful for the work that waiting did in me, and I am thankful that we are able to move forward in resting in our Father's plan for us. That is the best plan!

My After-Birth/Postpartum Experience: As soon as Elias was born, I sat down on the potty to let it catch anything that was still coming out of me. Eddie covered us with warm towels, and I looked down to see the umbilical cord turning white. Then it occurred to me that at any moment the placenta could fall into the toilet. That made me very nervous and I asked my hubby to grab the bowl I had planned to birth the placenta into. I panicked and asked him to grab the clamp and scissors instead, quickly. We had only one clamp, so he put it on baby's side of cord, the cord was very short in my opinion, less than 24 inches for sure. After Eddie cut the cord I held the maternal end of it up in the air because it was leaking blood and I wanted to be able to access how much I was bleeding without that adding to it. I have always had a tendency to bleed heavily, and I've never been given the chance to clot normally after a birth before.

I handed our son to hubby and he went to get the bowl. I got off the potty and kneeled down with one leg over the bowl and pushed the placenta out immediately. There was a trickle of blood that followed after the placenta. Eddie gave me a dose of shepherd's purse tincture (full dropper full) under my tongue. I just left the placenta there and walked to our bedroom, where there was a Chux pad already waiting for me, and pillows propped up in our bed. I had a slow trickle of blood coming out, so I started rubbing my abdomen. Then Eddie handed our son to me for skin to skin contact and to try and nurse him. He wasn't very interested, so I laid him in one arm, and we started using the breast pump while Eddie rubbed my abdomen. It was quite the sight. We had a whole postpartum kit for different scenarios and definitely for things we would try for bleeding. I am so glad now we had all those things in one place, because with just the two of us, it was hard to think what to do next with everything else going on.

Pumping my breasts definitely brought on stronger contractions, *VERY* painful. Hubby could feel uterus getting harder. It would rise just below my belly button on the right hand side of my abdomen with each contraction. Then we would take turns rubbing, being careful not to rub too hard.

I was filling up Chux pads pretty quickly and I could feel myself getting weaker as the time went on. Hubby replaced the warm towels and kept having me drink fluids.

I had purchased some cold peri pads, that we started using at this point. Eddie said I was really swollen down there, and it was a good idea to start the cold pads now. I wish I would have purchased more than 3 for the immediate postpartum. In the following days I was able to freeze washrags that were soaked in comfrey tea, but for the immediate those quick ones are very helpful.

Tried more shepherd's purse. I remembered that this causes clots, so we would rub my abdomen and a clot would come out followed by a gush of blood. This whole time my hubby was so calm though, and said that he still thought it was less blood loss than my last birth. We just needed to get it under control. I remembered to keep trying to empty my bladder, but at some point within the first hour after birth I started to get weaker and weaker and getting to the bathroom was getting harder, even though it's just steps outside of the bedroom.

I found it hard to breathe, I couldn't stand up straight, and finally I almost passed out. I felt my head get hot, and I sat down on the edge of the bathtub while hubby held baby and me up, and I put my head in his legs and just held on and told him I was about to black out. I never did fully, and when I felt I had the strength returned to bed with his help and my third dose of sheperd's purse, ½ dropper full. The bleeding was now starting to slow down and the shakes started for me. I took a dosage of Florodix liquid iron and drank a glass of orange juice. Hubby gave me Rescue Remedy when I started getting shaky, and that helped tons. I had two doses of that within the first hour. Our sweet baby boy finally latched on and ate for 10 minutes within the first hour of being born, and then fell asleep peacefully.

The first 24 hours were the hardest for me. I didn't walk on my own, thanking God for Eddie and the strength he provided physically and emotionally.

The position and the size of Elias, we believe, have caused my pubic bones and hip bones to feel like they were hit by a bus. The bones are still sore 9 days postpartum. I may have torn, but we aren't doing anything other than keeping legs together and resting. I did get a hemorrhoid from pushing, but it's going away now. I have had a normal BM everyday that doesn't hurt, so I know my perineum is intact. My bladder could use more muscle for sure. Working on one Kegel at a time.

Milk came in without a problem before the end of day 2. Latching on and breastfeeding is going great. On day 5 post birth, I lost a huge blood clot, and I haven't had much bleeding since. I have never stopped bleeding this soon, so I worry about that, naturally. Anything different or out of 'my' ordinary, causes me to question. My Eddie said to just be thankful, I don't have any symptoms of anything retained, and it's a good sign I'm resting and healing.

I've had one night of bad chills and sweating, but nothing since that night. I am taking Echinacea everyday, and keeping up on my vitamins.

He's my first baby to not get jaundice, and he doesn't snort or make those wet gurgle noises. His breathing has been so quiet and clear from the moment hubby laid him on my chest. This is very new to me. He is much more alert, and coos at us already. I guess letting them bake until they are ready to be born really does make a big difference in the way they behave.

*My Journey Through Birth by Danielle:*

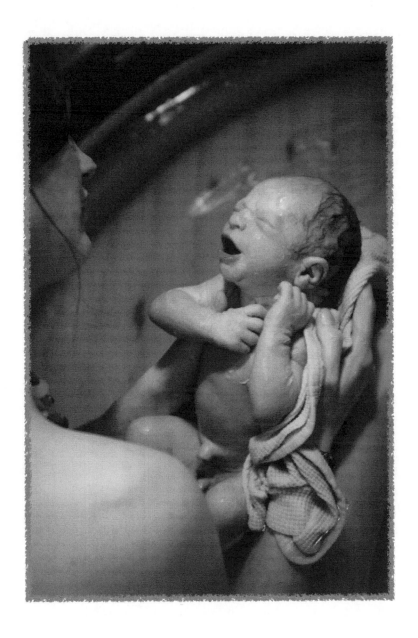

We had been seeing a midwife and her apprentice out of Salem for this pregnancy. We came up with the EDD of February 10th, 2008, however, this little one decided to hang out a little longer. With March right around the corner and both our midwife (Pamela) and her apprentice leaving Oregon in a couple of days, I was really hoping our baby would come soon.

The morning of March 4th, Pamela and I talked about our options for birth ( she was leaving the next day). We decided to try some castor oil. If my body was ready for labor it could help move things along. I had been having contractions on and off for a few days but nothing would come of them. I would rest and they would stop. So I went and got the castor oil. When we got home I took the kids for a long walk. I really wanted our midwife to be at the birth. Our last midwife couldn't make it due to being sick. We got her back up Dr., who we met only once. When we got back from the walk, we all took a nap. I woke up with more of the same contractions that I have been having the past few days. I took the castor oil around 1:30 PM and went about our afternoon. Around 5:00 PM, I had to use the bathroom and still feeling the same as before so not sure if the oil really worked.

I made dinner, called Nick, my husband, to see if he was on his way home from work. Between 5 and 7 I was still not feeling like I was in labor. Around 7:30 PM, I said to Nick I think that this might be it. I called Pamela at 7:45 PM to let her know that I thought I was in labor. Contractions were 5-7 minutes apart. She said to call her back when they are closer together or if I just wanted her to be there. I called my good friend Brett at 8:00 PM to let her know labor started and to come when she was ready. By the time I was off the phone with her it was feeling like the real thing. We are going to have our baby!! I had Nick call Pamela right back, she's on her way.

As I waited for Pamela and friends to arrive , I rode the waves of labor. Brett got to the house around 8:15 PM. I was so into labor by then I just gave her a smile. Nick was busy keeping the older two busy. Around 8:30 PM, he lit a candle and put it on the front porch so everyone could find their way. Two more friends arrived shortly after. I tried sitting on the birth ball but walking around felt much better. From here till birth went so fast that I had no sense of time.

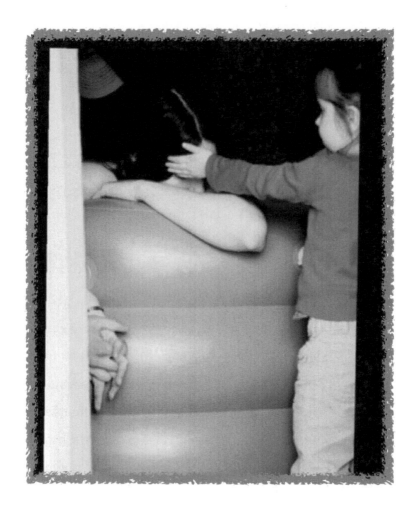

After walking a while I was ready to try out the tub, so Nick got on
filling it up. I stood over the birth tub as it was filling and the
sound of the water was so soothing. All of the sudden, I felt like I
needed to use the bathroom. Brett went with me just in case it was
the baby. I don't know why, but it felt nice to just sit on the toilet.
It was neither. I went in to the living room and danced in circles,

and that felt nice. I had the feeling that this is what it felt like right before my daughter was born. We just got started, so how could this be!?

The tub was as full as it was going to get; the hot water ran out. I didn't mind at that point. I just wanted in! At first, I was not so sure if I liked it or not that things were moving fast. This baby wanted to be born. After I relaxed, it was wonderful! I labored the rest of the time on my knees leaning over the side of the tub. I had so many wonderful people supporting me, including my almost three year old daughter who was giving me lots of loving hugs and kisses through out labor.

I asked Brett to call and see how far away Pamela was from the house. About 15 minutes. With the next contraction, I felt the baby move down into the birth canal. I reached inside and felt the bag of water. Then it hit me; the urge to push. This baby was not waiting. I gave a little push and the bag of water popped. It was such a cool feeling since my other two labors the waters were broken for me. With the next contraction, the baby's head was crowning and I said, in this deep voice, that I have never heard before, 'the baby is coming' and the head was out. Then the body shot out like a rocket, as my 6 year old described.

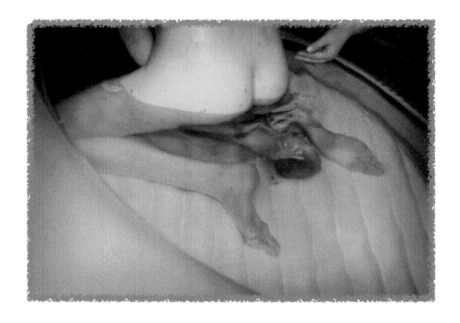

I pulled my baby through my legs and unwrapped the cord from his arm. What a beautiful baby. I was in bliss! I sobbed and thanked every one for there wonderful support. My son said, 'Well, mom, is it a boy or girl?' With it all happening so fast, I didn't even look. I looked down and it was an *ALDER!!* He was so, so excited to have a baby brother!

I stood up and delivered the placenta. I got comfortable on the bed to nurse him and he took to breastfeeding really well. He was born five minutes before Pamela arrived at the house. She checked us both out, and we were both good to go.

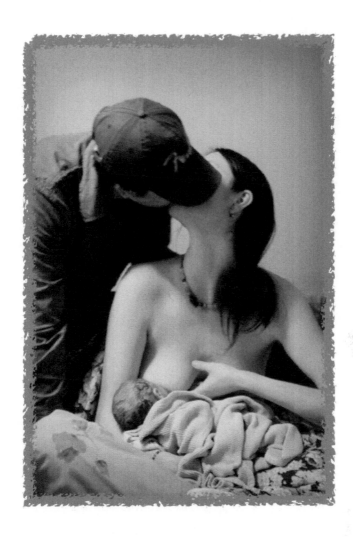

Alder James was born at 9:03 PM weighing 7lbs 13oz. I was so empowered by his birth. I had no one checking for dilation. No one telling me I was "ready" to push or not to push. I surrendered to the power of labor letting my body lead the way. It was very fast and intense and worth every second of it. Thank you to everyone who was involved in my pregnancy and his birth.

# My Journey Through Birth by Lisa:

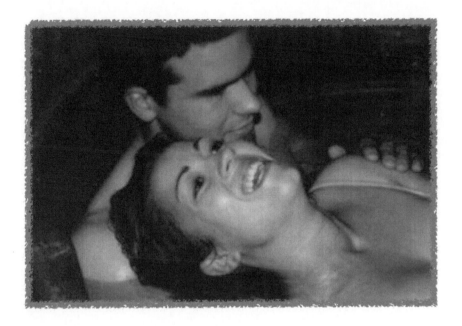

From my first time giving birth at age eighteen, I had always held a strong belief in natural labor and childbirth. Birth is a wonderful, empowering event that every woman is capable of experiencing. I would not dream of surrendering this rite of passage to drugs or hospital procedures. Now that I am pregnant with my fourth child, my love for labor and childbirth continues to grow. However, prior to the home-birth of my third child, giving birth outside of a hospital was an unknown realm to me.

While the births of all three of my children have been unique, sacred experiences, I wish to focus on the birth of my third child. The birth of Noah, may be a way to open the door for women who are considering birthing at home. Noah was born in the water on February 17, 2007 in the comfort of our own bedroom. The first hands to caress his tiny head were mine followed by my husband's, then my daughter's. There is something magical about being able to reach down and deliver your own child, and my wish is for every mother to have this opportunity.

In addition to the beauty of the birth itself, laboring in my own home was a comfort unsurpassed by any hospital or birthing center around the world. Aside from the obvious benefits such as not having to deal with hospital staff, infant seats, paperwork, middle-of-the-night visits from nurses and such, being at home enabled my labor to progress in a very comfortable manner. I don't think I really even realized I was in active labor until I reached the transition phase. Up until that point, I had been listening to relaxing C.D.s, sitting on my birthing ball, visiting with my husband and children, and making phone calls to distant family members. I hope that the smile on my face in these pictures is a telltale sign of the joy and ease I felt bringing Noah into the world!

Finally, there is nothing like having your own bed for your recovery bed. Noah was born at 10:37 PM. Shortly after midnight the three of us (my husband, myself, and Noah,) were snuggled

172

into bed, the bedroom was clean, laundry was washing, and the midwives were quietly letting themselves out the front door. I will never forget that moment, looking down at Noah while he nursed and my husband as he slept, thinking, "That's it? I just gave birth two hours ago and now I am left alone with my beautiful, healthy baby boy beside me in my own bed? Wow, that was too easy." However, maybe 'natural' would be a better word to describe the feeling. Yes, after six years and three children, I had finally obtained my 'natural' birth.

Words cannot describe the special spirit that permeated our home those first few days after Noah's birth. I was very protective of my home, a sanctuary for our littlest one. I kept visitors to a minimum, as I did not want any part of the "world" to interrupt these precious first days together. My other two children accepted Noah right away, and the time we spent bonding as a family is very memorable.

Doctors and hospitals have their place, but to every woman who is capable and willing to have her baby at home, I would highly endorse it. I am forever faithful to home birth, and I would never turn back. To any woman who knows what her body can do and is considering home birth, I would say that home birth is birth the way nature intended. It takes childbirth back to its roots. Bringing a child into the world is a sacred experience any way you look at it, but birthing at home enables the child and his or her family to reap all the blessings that come with the miracle of birth.

## Kaitlyn's Birth:

My due date was January 10th, 2008. This was the day of Jacob's 4th birthday. I knew she would come sooner. At least I hoped. On Saturday the 5th, I took the kids on a 3 mile bike ride, while I pushed Noah in the jogger stroller. We went up some long, steep hills. It was very windy and foggy that day, and the walk was quite strenuous. Later that afternoon, Lisa Perillo came over to visit, and as we were talking in the kitchen, I paused for a couple of moderately strong contractions. Looking back, that was the moment I knew pre-labor had begun. Later in the evening, I reverted to nesting mode and frantically began laundry (I needed clean towels and underwear!). I finished right around midnight, then went to bed.

On Sunday, we went to church as usual, and in Relief Society I shifted in my chair. I was now feeling the contractions in my lower back. I bore my testimony in Sacrament Meeting, and later on a couple of women told me, "You're going to have your baby soon!" Little did they know how soon. We put the kids to bed, and Forrest wanted to stay up a little later with me. However, I felt tired, and part of me knew that if I didn't go to bed, I'd pay for it. We lay down around 10:00 PM.

Right around midnight, I awoke to a scene I will never forget. Ashlee and Jacob were at my bedside, telling me they had both just thrown up. I jumped up and followed them both into the bathroom. Ashlee was getting sick, again, and Jacob was just standing there crying. It was at that moment that I noticed my first real labor contraction. My first thought was, you've got to be kidding! I stripped the kids of their clothes, threw their blankets into the washer, and tucked them back into bed. I lay back down in bed and tried to fall back to sleep, but was soon awakened again by the sound of feet scrambling to the bathroom. This continued throughout the night, intermingled with contractions spaced 5-10 minutes apart, strong enough to keep me from falling back to sleep. At one point, out of sheer desperation, I thought, I am going to go to the hospital and have this baby!

Around 5:00 AM I decided to make a decision. I got up, went downstairs, and called my mom. She answered, and I said through tears, "Mom, I'm in labor and the kids are throwing up. I need you, I can't do this alone." She told me she'd be right over.

After that, I came upstairs and woke Forrest. I will never forget how he sat up, fully awake and energized, and said with a smile, "We are going to have our baby today." Seeing him so confident and excited gave me renewed strength. It was then that I reaffirmed to myself, okay, I can do this. We went downstairs together and I called Marlene. She answered, sleepily, and I told her I'd been having contractions five minutes apart. By this time it was about 5:30 AM. She asked if I felt like I wanted them to come right now, and I said, "I don't know, maybe within an hour." After I hung up, I had one more contraction in the living room with Forrest holding me, and when it was over I said, "Call Marlene back and tell her to come sooner than later!"

Marlene, Kaleem, and my mom all arrived around 6:00 AM. I had had a few contractions sitting on the bed, and now I was in the bathroom, kneeling over the toilet. Psychosomatically, I was feeling slightly nauseated at the peak of each contraction. At one point I actually gagged into the toilet like I was going to get sick, but I think it was just that I was tired (and paranoid from cleaning up after the kids all night.) Marlene asked if I wanted them to set up the birthing tub. I wasn't sure how far along I was, and I didn't want the water to get cold. She said, "Let's check you and see." I stood up, and Kaleem knelt down and listened to the baby's heartbeat with the Doppler. Then I lay down on the bed for Marlene to check my cervix. This was quick and painless, and she reported, "Well, you're at about a 7." I don't think I responded quite as excitedly as she expected me to, probably because of my anxious anticipation of transition. I knew all too well what lay ahead.

She immediately began filling up the tub at the foot of our bed, and I resumed my place on the bathroom floor, resting my head on a folded towel placed on the toilet seat. For this labor, I felt very inclined to be in a kneeling position. Never once did I lie down. I could feel Kaitlyn's head exerting pressure with each contraction, as her head was positioned very low, and to lie down would've been counterproductive. Staying in an upright position gave me a feeling of control. I moved over to my bedside and had a few more contractions. After leaving the bathroom, I remember walking over towards the tub, longing to climb in, and seeing it only several inches full. Marlene stated, "I'm filling it as fast as I can." At this point, my mom, who had left the room, appeared in the doorway and stated that someone was here to see me. It was Brother Reed and Brother Madsen, whom Forrest had called earlier to give me a blessing. I told my mom to tell them it was too late, and to send them away. They came up anyways, feeling inclined to give the blessing. As soon as I saw them entering the room, I said, "Make it quick!" Miraculously, my contractions ceased while they were giving the blessing (or their timing was impeccable,) and no sooner did they descend the stairs than I had a pushing-urge contraction. I was being rather vocal, and I suddenly felt an overwhelming urge to take all my clothes off. I think this was my body's way of saying, get ready, the baby's coming!

The tub was finally ready, and Forrest and I climbed in together. Someone brought Ashlee and Jacob into our room and set them on the foot of the bed, overlooking the birth tub. My water had not yet broken and I knew Kaitlyn's head was right there, but I had not yet mustered up the strength to begin pushing. I reached in to break my bag of waters, but was unable. Marlene said she would try to get it, but then said that her head was ready to come out, and there was no need to break the water. Within a couple of good pushes, her head came out, to which I responded, "Oh, thank goodness." I knew the hard part was over, and relief flooded my exhausted body. The next contraction brought the rest of her body out, and to the surprise of us all, the bag of waters was still intact! Marlene told us that this was a sign of luck across all cultures. I reached down and lifted her slippery little body out of the water and onto my chest, and Marlene gently peeled the membranes over her head and off her body. We sat there in the water admiring our little princess, and then climbed into bed after the placenta was delivered.

The first thing I noticed about Kaitlyn was her long feet! She surprised me by being even smaller than her brother at 6 lbs. 12oz. Someone brought Noah into the room, and we all cozied up in bed together as the morning light began to come in through the window. She had been born at 7:21 AM.

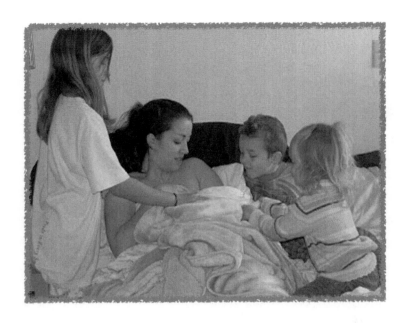

The midwives continued on with their usual routine of cleaning up, starting laundry, and making tea. All my fears of the previous night had vanished as we relished in the love and spirit that our precious baby girl had brought into our home.

My love for home-birth was rekindled all over again! I know that things played out the way they did for a reason, for had the kids not been sick, I may not have called my mom until after the birth. She was in awe over the experience, and I was grateful to have her there. Kaitlyn's birth was nothing short of a miracle, as were the births of all my children. I am so amazed by this wonderful and sacred power that Heavenly Father has given to women, and I wouldn't trade the experience, or the children I've been blessed with, for anything in the world.

I get out of the shower and take out my little baby bathtub so I can stand over it and catch my baby. The phone rings. For some reason I answer it....

I return to the bathtub and straddle it. I am not pushing. This baby is coming out on her own. I look down and see a face covered by a thin film. The baby is still in the water bag. It breaks as she slides into my hands. She looks into my eyes as her body emerges. I am elated. There is no one else in the world - only she and I. She is the most beautiful gift I have ever received. I hold her close and cry. I have climbed the mountain. I have reached the top and been rewarded beyond my wildest dreams!

Within minutes the placenta slips out as I squat over the bathtub. I tie and cut her cord and put her in a baby seat. Suddenly I'm exhausted. I lay down on the couch and begin to hear strange, lovely sounds - ocean waves gently crashing on the shore, and wind chimes - but we are a thousand miles from the sea and there is no wind today. I am in ecstasy.

- *Laura Shanley,* a free-lance writer, birth consultant, speaker, poet, author of the book *Unassisted Childbirth,* and owner of Bornfree Bookshop.

## I Believe...by Laura Shanley

I Believe.....

That birth is inherently safe. The same loving, intelligent consciousness (All That Is, Goddess, God, Nature) that knows how to grow an egg and a sperm into a human being, knows how to get it out. Our job is simply to relax and trust. Birth is not a function of the conscious mind any more than digestion is.

I Believe.....

That the problems women sometimes encounter in birth can be traced to three main causes:

Poverty - lack of food and poor living conditions

Outside interference - doctors and sometimes midwives poking, prodding, testing, drugging, cutting, etc.

Inside interference - primarily fear which triggers the fight/flight response and shuts down labor, but also shame and guilt

When these factors are eliminated, most women can give birth easily, either alone or with friends and family.

I Believe.....

That our bodies and our babies are responsive to our thoughts. The best way to ensure a good pregnancy and birth is to think positively, face and overcome our fears, and believe in our own abilities.

# Trust and Transformation

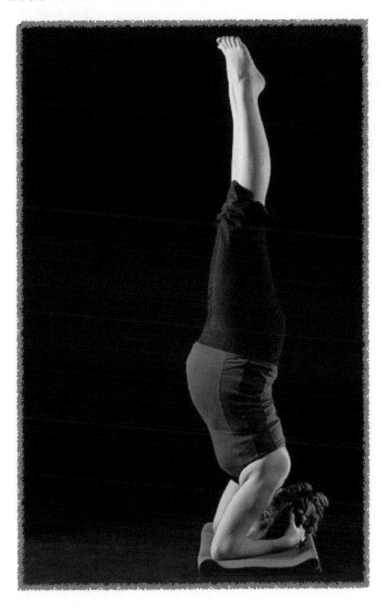

This is a time unlike no other in a woman's life. This is a time unlike no other in the father's life. The birthing of a child will bring up fears and concerns that you may have never known were there. When explored, respected and released, a woman and a man may more fully and safely experience pregnancy, labor, birth and parenting the way it is meant to be. A beautiful, trustworthy process that will transform you into a truer reflection of yourself.

In the end, you will be the author of your birth stories. Either by action or non-action. Either by being an active writer or a non-active observer of the story. This is your body, your baby and your story. Be empowered and let it transform you. Let the beauty of the process unfold you and mold you into the woman and man you are to become. The process of pregnancy shapes you for mothering and how you are as a mother is greatly a product of the process of your pregnancy, labor and birth.

I offer you blessings of joy, love, growth, empowerment and transformation during this journey and may you love the woman and man that you become and the babies that you birth.
###
Thank you for reading my book. If you enjoyed it, won't you please take a moment to leave me a review at your favorite retailer? Remember that there is a print version which I hand mail out from my home. You can always find this book thru www.taralmcguire.com .

THANKS!

Tara McGuire

# Resources

Here is a list of resources that can assist you in your journey.

•*Creating a Joyful Birth Experience*: Developing a Partnership with Your Unborn Child for Healthy Pregnancy, Labor, and Early Parenting by Lucia Capacchione & Sandra Bardsley

•*Unassisted Childbirth* by Laura Kaplan Shanley

•*Birthing from Within:* An Extra-Ordinary Guide to Childbirth Preparation by Pam England & Rob Horowitz

•*Pushed*: The Painful Truth About Childbirth and Modern Maternity Care by Jennifer Block

•Midwifery Today at midwiferytoday.com

•Birth Works© Inc. at www.birthworks.org

•Ryan Kackley, N.L.P. C.Ht. E.F.T, *Celt System* Founder, Relationship Consulting.  www.celtsystem.com  503-999-7685

# About The Author

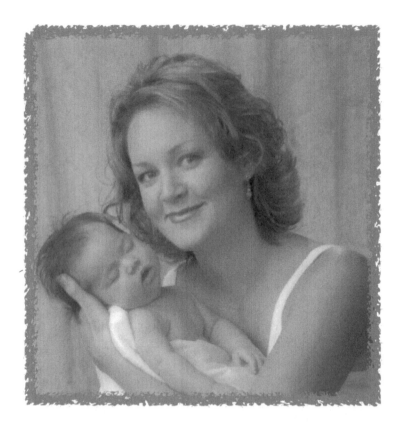

Tara L. McGuire is a home-schooling mother of four. She works mostly from home as a writer and advocate/speaker of the topics of personal development and empowerment. Tara also is marketing director and studio manager for Indigo Yoga Studios and Indigo Wellness Center. As a yoga instructor of Hatha yoga, she also enjoys combining her back ground as a child birth educator with her skills as a yoga instructor to offer a creative body/mind/spirit prenatal class.

In addition to these endeavors, Tara is a business consultant and web designer, offering a holistic approach to business development. All of these avenues give Tara the ability to do the two things that she loves: be with her children and influence the growth and prosperity in people's lives.

Tara's purpose and mission statement:
*The purpose of my life is to experience joy and abundance by inspiring and empowering individuals to live a richer and more meaningful life.*

Connect with me:

www.facebook.com/birthunhindered
www.taralmcguire.com

10644700R00105

Printed in Great Britain
by Amazon.co.uk, Ltd.,
Marston Gate.